the
RHODIOLA
REVOLUTION

the

RHODIOLA
REVOLUTION

TRANSFORM YOUR HEALTH WITH THE
HERBAL BREAKTHROUGH OF THE 21ST CENTURY

RICHARD P. BROWN, M.D., *and*
PATRICIA L. GERBARG, M.D.
with Barbara Graham

RODALE

© 2004 by Richard P. Brown, M.D., and Patricia L. Gerbarg, M.D.

First published 2004
First published in paperback 2005

Book design by Christopher Rhoads

Cover illustration courtesy of the LuEsther T. Matz Library
of the New York Botanical Garden, Bronx, New York

Library of Congress Cataloging-in-Publication Data

Brown, Richard P.
    The rhodiola revolution : transform your health with the herbal breakthrough of the 21st
century / Richard P. Brown and Patricia L. Gerbarg, with Barbara Graham.
        p.   cm.
    Includes bibliographical references and index.
    ISBN-13 978–1–57954–924–4 hardcover
    ISBN-10 1–57954–924–1 hardcover
    ISBN-13 978–1–59486–294–6 paperback
    ISBN-10 1–59486–294–X paperback
    1. Roseroot—Therapeutic use.   I. Gerbarg, Patricia L.   II. Graham, Barbara.   III. Title.
RM666.R586B767   2004
615'.32372—dc22   2004003901

Distributed to the trade by Holtzbrinck Publishers

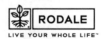

IN LOVING MEMORY OF OUR PARENTS

Dr. David S. Gerbarg

Colonel Gerhard Brown

Marie Brown

TO THE PARENTS WHO ARE STILL WITH US

Dorothy Gerbarg-Barzin

Richard Barzin

TO OUR WONDERFUL CHILDREN

Laura, Joshua, and David

TO THE WISDOM OF OUR TEACHERS

Sri Sri Ravi Shankar

Sensei Imaizumi

CONTENTS

PART I:
RHODIOLA ROSEA
AND THE HUMAN ENERGY CRISIS

PART II:
WHAT *RHODIOLA ROSEA*
CAN DO FOR YOU

PART III:

ENERGIZED FOR LIFE

FOREWORD

This book is a most welcome addition to the growing body of literature on herbs and phytomedicines. In the past few decades, interest in herbs and phytomedicinal products has grown, not only in the United States but also throughout the world. In recent years, some of this interest has focused on *Rhodiola rosea.*

All too often, when consumers and health professionals think about herbs, the ones that come to mind are the most popular in the marketplace—what I sometimes endearingly refer to as the "usual suspects." These include aloe vera, black cohosh, echinacea, garlic, ginger, ginkgo, ginseng, saw palmetto, St. John's wort, and valerian, among numerous others. Most of these herbs have achieved their prominence in the marketplace because they have been the subjects of the most clinical research.

The past 10 to 20 years have witnessed an explosion in the scientific study of herbal formulations. Until very recently, much of this research took place in western Europe—particularly in Germany, where a unique regulatory system evaluates the safety and indications of herbs sold in pharmacies, approving about 200 of them as nonprescription medicines. Other countries involved in extensive herbal research include China, Japan, India, and Russia. Very few of the studies from Russia and the former Soviet Union had been available in the West because they had not been translated into English, the predominant international language of science and medicine.

This is one of the major reasons why the West has remained largely unaware of the increasingly impressive health benefits of *Rhodiola rosea,* sometimes called Arctic root or golden root. Most of the research occurred in Russia and appeared in Russian medical journals. The data from many of these studies have been under wraps until recently, when they began to appear in limited venues.

At least three modern, well-designed, controlled clinical trials on the adaptogenic properties of *Rhodiola rosea* have been published in *Phytomedicine,* a leading English-language journal on the science of herbs and medicinal plants. The results of these trials strongly support the safety and efficacy of *Rhodiola rosea.* Unfortunately, such trials need to appear in leading medical journals before the conventional medical community will take notice of the potential applications of *Rhodiola rosea* in modern clinical practice. Publication in major medical journals also could increase media coverage of herbs like *Rhodiola rosea* and thus promote their inclusion in a rational regimen of dietary supplementation for millions of consumers who are looking for ways to increase energy, reduce stress, and optimize their well-being.

Fortunately, the literature documenting the health benefits of *Rhodiola rosea* has been comprehensively and painstakingly reviewed by two medical experts who are able to present a clear, cogent, and concise case for the appropriate incorporation of *Rhodiola rosea* into both medical practice and consumer self-care. I first met Dr. Dick Brown and Dr. Pat Gerbarg over the Internet, via a series of e-mails. They had prepared an extensive monograph on *Rhodiola rosea* for the American Botanical Council's peer-reviewed herbal medicine journal *HerbalGram* (www.herbalgram.org), of which I am the editor. Over the ensuing months, I worked with them to develop the manuscript into what became the first authoritative and comprehensive English-language review of the clinical and pharmacological literature about this fascinating herb.

Normally, I am not one to hype the next "superherb." Too often, the U.S. herb market has been characterized by sharp peaks in interest based on the introduction of a "new" herb or the "latest miracle discovery." (This market dynamic also is true for nonherbal dietary supplements.) But when I was interviewed for a one-page story that appeared in the February 3, 2003, issue of *Newsweek* magazine, I did say that *Rhodiola rosea* might become the next "herbal superstar." I continue to believe this, for several reasons.

First and foremost, the herb is extremely safe. Based on centuries of use—going back almost 2,000 years to its documented tradition as a remedy in classic Greek medicine—plus numerous animal and human clinical studies, *Rhodiola rosea* has demonstrated a high degree of safety. It is not known to produce any serious adverse effects and few, if any, minor side effects.

Second, as this book clearly demonstrates, *Rhodiola rosea* has a wide array of documented health benefits, from its established role in building energy and stamina to its potential in helping stabilize depressive moods. The research to support each benefit has been carefully detailed by Dr. Brown and Dr. Gerbarg.

Third, an impressive body of scientific literature supports the traditional and modern applications of *Rhodiola rosea*. Often scientists and health professionals are not satisfied with the level of clinical research on many herbs—and, in general, I tend to agree with them. That is, I would prefer to see much more research on most herbs. But with regard to *Rhodiola rosea*, the published studies so far show the herb to be useful for physical and mental performance under stress, energy enhancement, heart health, immune defense, hormone balance, and weight loss.

Finally, *Rhodiola rosea* is agriculturally sustainable. There is a growing sense of urgency among environmental biologists and other scientists in similar fields, as well as among responsible members of the herbal industry, that the continued worldwide demand for herbal

medicines could have a deleterious impact on native plant populations. This legitimate concern is particularly relevant to herbs like
Rhodiola rosea, whose desired medicinal part is the root. To harvest
the root, the entire plant must be destroyed. Fortunately, forward-
thinking farmers and entrepreneurs in various parts of Russia, some
former Soviet republics, and Scandinavia are developing commercial
Rhodiola rosea farms, where they can cultivate high-quality root material without putting further pressure on wild stands of the herb. As
a bonus, this practice will help establish a viable new industry in
countries in urgent need of economic development.

In choosing this book for your personal library, you're getting authoritative, reliable information from two medical experts who not
only understand the professional literature but also have used adaptogens like *Rhodiola rosea* personally and in their professional practices. The term *adaptogen* is highly appropriate to describe the actions
of a group of herbs for which we in the West have few other words,
except perhaps the less adequate *tonic. Adaptogen* was coined in the
late 1940s by Soviet pharmacologists who were studying the actions
of the legendary Asian ginseng root (*Panax ginseng).* Adaptogens, as
this excellent book explains, are safe, natural substances that support
an organism in responding to various stressors, whether heat, cold, fatigue, emotional upset, or—in the case of *Rhodiola rosea*—prolonged
periods of weightlessness and the extreme stresses of spaceflight.

This book will help to bridge the knowledge gap that exists about
the safety and potential health benefits of *Rhodiola rosea.* I consider
it an essential resource for consumers and health professionals alike.

—*Mark Blumenthal*
Founder and executive director,
American Botanical Council
Editor, HerbalGram

ACKNOWLEDGMENTS

This book never could have been written without the help of many friends and colleagues. More than anyone else, Dr. Zakir Ramazanov deserves credit for introducing us to *Rhodiola rosea* and for his tireless efforts to recover and translate many original research documents from the former Soviet Union and other countries. We cannot thank Zakir enough for the generosity with which he has shared his time, his scientific knowledge, and his friendship and for taking Dick to subarctic mountain peaks to find the most potent wild herbs.

We also want to acknowledge the contributions of our patients, who allowed us to borrow from their own medical histories to create the case studies we present in this book. Although we have changed names and other identifying information to protect privacy, all of the cases are based on real people. They've shared parts of their personal stories in the best spirit of giving because they understand the importance of spreading the word about a new treatment like *Rhodiola rosea*, which might help others as it has helped them overcome health problems and lead happier, more fulfilling lives. We recognize their courage in their determination to not let sickness defeat them and in their willingness to trust and to try something new.

We are deeply grateful to Sri Sri Ravi Shankar and the teachers of the Art of Living Foundation for showing us how to accept the present moment as it is, the importance of belonging to everyone, the gift of silence, and the ways to achieve a calm, clear mind through Sudarshan Kriya Yoga and meditation.

Our sincere gratitude goes to our dear colleagues Dr. Rena Appel, Dr. Sharon Sageman, Dr. Charles Silverstein, and Stephanie Smith, R.N., for sharing their experiences with *Rhodiola rosea* in the course of their clinical practices. We also drew upon scientific information provided by Dr. Patricia K. Eagon, Dr. George Wikman, Chris Kilham, and the Swedish Herbal Institute. Mark Blumenthal's comments on our review of *Rhodiola rosea* for the American Botanical Council's magazine, *HerbalGram*, helped to sharpen the focus of our core scientific material. Laura Braslow provided invaluable assistance in editing and preparing our drafts. And Dr. Beth Abrams provided the verse that ends our book on such a graceful note.

Our most affectionate thanks go to our families for their support and encouragement. Our children gave us the most honest and blunt criticisms, including "No! For my sake, please, no!" and "Ugh!" Thanks to their careful and tasteful editing, our readers have been spared our worst efforts.

Finally, we would like to thank Tami Booth, Susan Berg, and the staff of Rodale Women's Health Books, who have poured their knowledge, skills, and creative talents into making this book a reality.

—*Dick and Pat*

I thank Joy Harris for bringing this project to me; Mark Matousek for recommending me; Tami Booth and Susan Berg for their invaluable assistance in helping to shape this book; Audrey Ferber for patiently standing by while I (often noisily) worked my way through the science; my husband, Hugh Delehanty, for cheerfully enduring five months of obsession with a previously obscure herb; and my son, Clay McLachlan, for just being.

—*Barbara*

Impressions of a REMARKABLE HERB

The inspiration for this book began with a serendipitous chain of events that could not have been timelier. Little did we know when we first heard about a mysterious herb called *Rhodiola rosea* that it would have such a profound effect on our own health, as well as the health of our patients, family members, friends, and colleagues.

PAT'S STORY

In the early 1990s, we got our first puppy. Because we live in an area that's heavily populated with deer, it wasn't long before Rocky started bringing deer ticks into the house. Each day I checked him carefully and removed the tiny pests. I wanted to make sure that none of my three children got bitten or developed Lyme disease.

After a few months of this, I noticed some discomfort in my joints. I didn't pay much attention to it at the time because I had a history of back pain and I never got the telltale rash that indicates a tick bite.

But over the course of the next year, the pain intensified, spreading from my joints into my tendons and muscles.

I consulted doctors and had every possible test—MRIs, CAT scans, blood workups, spinal taps, and nerve conduction studies. Invariably, the results were normal. Even when I told the story about the dog and the ticks, my doctors insisted that I couldn't possibly have Lyme disease because my blood and spinal fluid showed no trace of it.

In fact, some of the specialists whom I consulted believed that there was no basis for my pain. That was a good lesson for me. I learned what it's like to be a patient with a doctor who doesn't really believe that the person is ill. When I was sick, my view of the medical profession changed, as did my faith in conventional medicine, which I thought had all the answers.

All the while, I was losing my strength, as well as my energy, as the pain kept getting worse. I couldn't use my hands for much of anything. They hurt so much that even the simplest activity, like brushing my teeth, was excruciating. My children became my hands. They washed the dishes. Laura, who was a teenager, handled my correspondence and wrote checks for me. I spent a lot of time lying flat, with ice packs or heat packs on my joints, waiting for the pain to subside. Any movement was unbearable.

Walking became a problem, too. I had the shuffling gait of a woman in her eighties, even though I was only in my forties. It took everything inside me just to get from the house to the car, and from the car up the stairs to my office.

Of course, I tried many different medications, but none of them helped. As the months and years went by, I coped by reducing my level of activity, including the number of hours I saw patients. Because I was having trouble sitting, I got in the habit of lying on the couch during our sessions. I also taught my patients how to write their own prescriptions, which I'd "sign" with a rubber stamp of my name. We

joked that mine was the only office where the patients wrote the prescriptions while the psychiatrist lay on the couch.

During this time, the thing that was hardest for me was not being
able to dance. My husband, Dick, and I love ballroom dancing. We'd
begun entering competitions and even winning some. After I got sick,
I couldn't dance. I adjusted to every other loss, but not this one.
Thankfully, we had a wonderful teacher who adapted the steps so I
could just kind of shuffle around and wave my arms.

The most touching moment came when I went with my son Josh to
visit colleges. At one of the schools, we had to park at the bottom of
a hill and climb several flights of concrete steps to reach the campus.
I told my son, "Josh, there's no way I can get up those stairs. You go
without me." Well, he picked me up and carried me not only to the
top of the hill but right to the building where his interview was. This
happened again and again: My legs would give out—as we were visiting schools or attending family events—and Josh would pick me up
and carry me. In one way, being sick was hard because I didn't want
to burden my children. Yet in another way, it was a blessing because
I could see how my children were becoming more aware and more
compassionate and considerate of others.

Eventually, Dick—who's a psychopharmacologist and an expert in
alternative medicine—ran into a colleague with symptoms similar to
mine. This doctor had been helped by a specialist in infectious diseases, so we made an appointment. The specialist ordered a PET
(positron-emission tomography) scan, which found reduced bloodflow to several areas of my brain, caused by vasculitis, an inflammation of the blood vessels. This made sense because I had started losing
my memory and was having increasing difficulty with balance. It was
very frightening.

The doctor suggested that the most likely cause of my symptoms was
an infection such as Lyme disease. Even though my tests came back

negative, he decided to treat me as though I had the disease. Later we learned that approximately 10 to 20 percent of Lyme disease cases may be seronegative. In other words, they don't show up in blood tests.

After an 8-month course of antibiotics, I showed some improvement in my mobility and strength, and I didn't have as much pain. All in all, I'd say I was about 25 percent better—which was a great relief. Still, I continued to have problems with my memory, concentration, and balance. Dick recommended supplements to support my nerve function while he searched for other things that might help even more.

DICK'S CHANCE "DISCOVERY"

One day a patient who had been struggling with depression came into my office feeling much cheerier. When I asked him what was going on, he told me about a little-known herb called rhodiola that he'd picked up in a health food store. I suspected his improved mood might be a placebo effect, so I didn't pay much attention to it. Then, a few months later, another patient came in with the same story.

Both of these men suffered from clinical depression and anxiety, and both had improved on antidepressants, though only to a limited extent. Suddenly they were reporting a much higher level of energy and a much greater capacity to experience pleasure. I decided to learn all that I could about rhodiola, which I hadn't heard of before.

Upon researching the market, I found only two preparations of the herb that looked reasonable. I wrote to one company and asked to see their studies. They directed me to an expert, a plant biochemist by the name of Dr. Zakir Ramazanov.

As it happened, Zakir not only had done research on *Rhodiola rosea*—the species of the plant that is most effective—but he also had recently moved to the United States and lived just an hour away from

Pat and me. On our first meeting soon after, I learned that his interest in the herb was not just professional. It had been the key to his recovery from severe post-traumatic stress disorder, which he'd developed after serving with the Soviet army during the war in Afghanistan.

Zakir gave me a stack of articles and studies, as well as a book, on the benefits of *Rhodiola rosea*, of which he was coauthor. I discovered that the herb—which grows at high altitudes in Siberia, the Republic of Georgia, and Scandinavia—calms the stress response system while increasing cellular energy. It also improves brain function and strengthens the immune system.

Right away I realized that *Rhodiola rosea* might help Pat. But before I recommend a new treatment to someone else, I like to try it on myself. So I started taking the herb to see how I'd feel. Almost immediately, my mind seemed clearer. I was more energetic and less stressed. After a few days, I noticed that I recovered from exercise more quickly. In fact, when I took *Rhodiola rosea*, I could work out harder without feeling as drained as before. And I didn't experience any side effects. So I gave the herb to Pat.

PAT'S REMARKABLE HEALING

Within 10 days of taking my first dose of *Rhodiola rosea*, my memory was on the rebound. I remember when I noticed a difference. It was a Sunday, and I felt the urge to play chess with my son David, then 14 years old. I had taught him to play when he was little, and since then he had become a competitive chess player on his high school team. I had given up the game during my illness because I couldn't concentrate long enough. On that Sunday, however, I felt up to the challenge. David reluctantly agreed, on one condition: I had to let him watch TV and do his math homework at the same time so he wouldn't be too bored.

We played, and to his surprise and dismay, I won. It was the first time in years that I'd mustered the mental ability to focus and remember the moves and strategies. It was just incredible. Of course, David won the rematch by paying close attention, but I put up a good fight.

Every day after that, it seemed, something else would come back that I thought I'd lost forever. One morning a couple of months after I started taking *Rhodiola rosea*, I jumped out of bed and began doing the rumba. Just like that. All the steps I'd learned that had been inaccessible to me during my illness were right there. I was thrilled to realize that someday I might really be able to dance again.

My mental function continued to improve, too. My thinking, which had become quite slow during my illness, returned to normal speed over several months. After years of struggling to "multitask," and forgetting what I was doing when I tried to focus on more than one thing at a time, I finally could take in more complex information. This is a critical skill when you have a job, a husband, three children, and a dog, as I do. You must be able to keep your bearings when so much is going on around you.

Over the next year, as my pain subsided, I gradually took on more patients. Now I can do things that I once took for granted—go for a walk, hold a pen, open a jar, drive a car. Best of all, I'm dancing with my husband again. I may not be quite as good as I once was, but when I dance, I really dance. Although I haven't recovered my full strength and I still need to be careful, I have my life back.

WHY WE WROTE THIS BOOK

Looking back, we believe that *Rhodiola rosea* probably rejuvenated the nerves that had been damaged by the reduced bloodflow to Pat's brain, in addition to energizing all the systems in her body. We were so surprised and grateful for her dramatic recovery that we decided to keep investigating the properties and benefits of this exceptional herb. Why hadn't we heard about it before?

We learned from Zakir that while *Rhodiola rosea* had been extensively studied in the former Soviet Union, most of the research had been concealed in classified documents. Since the fall of the regime in 1991, however, Zakir has devoted himself to recovering the original documents and painstakingly translating them. He generously made this substantial body of research available to us. We studied it closely and began recommending *Rhodiola rosea*, when appropriate, to patients, family members, friends, and colleagues—with overwhelmingly positive results. We have seen the herb make a real difference for hundreds of people suffering from fatigue, chronic stress, depression, memory and cognitive impairment, hormonal imbalances, and immune system dysfunction, as well as for healthy individuals seeking to improve their physical or mental endurance.

Such broad benefits may sound too good to be true. But as we'll explain in chapter 4, *Rhodiola rosea* is an adaptogen, a natural substance that acts on multiple systems of the body. Based on what we have seen, this hardy plant—with its powerful healing properties and very low toxicity—could help prevent or slow the progression of numerous diseases, while relieving suffering and vastly improving the quality of life for many people.

In the summer of 2003, Dick and Zakir had their own remarkable adventure with *Rhodiola rosea*.

Dick: We were climbing in the Sayan Mountains, the eastern continuation of the Altai range, on the northern border of Mongolia, searching for *Rhodiola rosea* growing in the wild. Our journey already had taken us 6,000 feet above sea level in just 3 hours. After scrambling for miles on slippery rocks in a cold glacial river, we followed our guide, Pavel, through subarctic terrain to an altitude of

10,000 feet. Our last hurdle was a 200-foot sheer rock cliff, which we somehow managed to scale. When we got to the other side, we were greeted by the bright golden flowers of *Rhodiola rosea* growing everywhere in the craggy walls of a ravine.

Exhausted, we carefully dug up some fresh roots, which we washed in a pure mountain stream, then sliced, boiled, and steeped in water. We quickly drank the hot, dark red tea. Even though each of us was familiar with *Rhodiola rosea*'s healing power, we weren't quite prepared for the blast of energy delivered by the herb. Within 15 minutes we felt strong enough to race down the mountain ahead of a gathering summer storm that might have swollen the river and trapped us in that remote, isolated ravine.

Because Pat and I have experienced the benefits of *Rhodiola rosea* firsthand, and because the herb remains relatively unknown in the West, our mission in writing this book is to share the scientific research—as well as our own clinical experience—with the general public, with physicians and other health care practitioners, and with research scientists. Our deepest hope is that the information presented here will inspire further investigation of *Rhodiola rosea* and be of as much benefit to our readers as it has been to us.

WHO WE ARE

Before we get too far into our exploration of *Rhodiola rosea*, we thought you might want to know a bit more about us and our qualifications to write a book like this. Allow us to introduce ourselves.

Dick: I'm an associate professor of clinical psychiatry at Columbia College of Physicians and Surgeons in New York City, with private practices in psychiatry and psychopharmacology in both Manhattan and upstate New York, where Pat and I live. For the last 15 years, I've specialized in working with patients who have complex psychiatric and medical histories and who often can't tolerate standard drug therapies. In addition to teaching and clinical work, I conduct research, having participated in numerous studies of psychiatric disorders. I'm also the author, with Teodora Bottiglieri, Ph.D., and Carol Colman, of *Stop Depression Now*, which presents a holistic approach to treating depression.

Although I received traditional medical training at Columbia University, throughout my career I've explored herbs and other alternative therapies as supplements to conventional drug treatments—but only when I find compelling scientific evidence to support their use. I won't recommend anything if the science behind it isn't solid. Just because a remedy is "natural" doesn't mean it's safe or effective. While some natural substances can heal, others do very little or, worse, cause serious damage. Knowing the difference can be a matter of life and death.

My lifelong interest in medicinal plants can be traced to my childhood in Kentucky, where I trailed my grandfather through the woods as he hunted for mushrooms and other plants with healing properties. Early on, I got the idea that things from nature can be very therapeutic for people. In fact, I learned from both sides of my family that we human beings have a powerful innate ability to heal. We just need to know how to activate it.

My positive clinical experience with *Rhodiola rosea*, SAM-e, and other natural substances has confirmed what I learned as a child. So has my personal experience. Because of my extremely demanding schedule, I depend on a daily regimen of yoga stretching, yoga breathing, and meditation—as well as aikido (a Japanese martial art), a healthful diet, and the use of *Rhodiola rosea*—to sustain my energy.

Pat: I'm an assistant clinical professor of psychiatry at New York Medical College in Valhalla. After graduating from Brown University, I trained at Harvard Medical School before completing my psychiatry residency at Beth Israel Hospital in Boston and my psychoanalytic training at the Boston Psychoanalytic Society and Institute. I have taught, supervised, and lectured on a wide range of topics in psychiatry, including stress, depression, and trauma. I maintain a private practice in upstate New York.

My appreciation of herbal medicine deepened considerably once I added *Rhodiola rosea* to my healing regimen during my long and difficult bout of Lyme disease. Since my recovery, I've gotten more and more interested in researching and writing about alternative and complementary medicine in psychiatry. Dick and I have been coauthors of numerous scientific articles and book chapters on the subject, including an in-depth article with Dr. Zakir Ramazanov on *Rhodiola rosea* for *HerbalGram*, and the chapter "Complementary and Alternative Treatments in Psychiatry" with Philip R. Muskin for the second edition of the textbook *Psychiatry*.

To maintain my energy reserves, I practice yoga stretching, yoga breathing, and meditation on a daily basis. In addition, I go for walks two or three times a day, and I maintain a healthy diet. Of course, I take *Rhodiola rosea* religiously, before breakfast and lunch.

A FINAL NOTE

Although we are great fans of *Rhodiola rosea*, we want to assure you that our interest in it is as scientists and physicians committed to providing our patients with the most effective treatments available, with the fewest side effects. We have no past, present, or prospective future financial interest in any product containing *Rhodiola rosea*, nor do we have a financial stake in any other supplement mentioned in this book.

Part I

Rhodiola rosea
and the
HUMAN
ENERGY
CRISIS

CHAPTER 1

Energy,
STRESS,
AND YOUR HEALTH

People are experiencing burnout like never before. It's easy to see why. Between cell phones, pagers, and instant messaging—not to mention job demands, family responsibilities, and a nonstop flow of obligations and commitments—we're on call 24/7. No matter how many tasks we cross off our to-do lists, they just keep getting longer. Then we must deal with the threats of terrorism; snipers; and SARS, West Nile virus, and other newly minted infectious diseases, which only fuel our anxiety levels. Just thinking about it all makes us toss and turn well into the night, compromising the sleep we so desperately need to replenish our dwindling energy reserves. We yawn and stumble through our days, feeling simultaneously tired and wired.

Does this sound familiar? If so, you may be one of the millions of Americans who chronically expend more energy than they have, someone whose energy reserves are almost always tapped out. This imbalance puts an enormous amount of stress on body and mind. It also is a leading cause of illness in the United States, where an estimated 80 percent of health problems stem from stress.

To get a clearer picture of how stress—or overspending your energy reserves—affects your health, imagine your body as a car battery that constantly uses energy without ever fully recharging. In other words, more energy is expended than replaced, so less and less juice is available over time. Eventually, the battery wears down, and the engine won't turn over.

We humans are similar. Everything we do, mentally as well as physically—from eating breakfast to planning the day's agenda to falling in love—burns energy. For this reason, we require a steady supply of energy in order to function well. These days, with so many pressures bearing down on us, our energy demands are greater than ever. And we need to store extra energy for use during unexpected crises.

We must replenish our energy reserves daily—ideally with more than we expend so that we always have an ample supply available for those times when we really need it. This may be what *Rhodiola rosea* does best.

RHODIOLA ROSEA:
NATURE'S PERFECT ENERGIZER

Rhodiola rosea is one of those rare substances that increase energy at the very source: our cells. For several decades, researchers have been examining the root of this remarkable herb, which grows wild at high altitudes in Siberia and other northern regions. Their conclusion? *Rhodiola rosea* actually boosts energy production in the cells of the major organ systems.

This power surge at the cellular level not only helps us manage stress with greater ease but also protects against disease and neutralizes environmental toxins. A growing body of evidence shows that *Rhodiola rosea* significantly improves physical and mental function, as well as the workings of the cardiovascular, immune, and neuroen-docrine systems. (The term *neuroendocrine* collectively refers to the neurological and endocrine systems. It's a product of current research that shows just how intimately connected these systems are.)

Our own positive clinical experience with the herb—as well as our colleagues'—is consistent with the research. We have found *Rhodiola rosea* to be extremely beneficial in treating depression, anxiety, chronic fatigue, neurological disorders, sexual dysfunction, and hor-monal imbalances. It also has helped many of our patients success-fully manage debilitating conditions such as cancer and Parkinson's disease—with few or, in most cases, no bothersome side effects.

We cannot emphasize the last point enough. By the time they seek our counsel, many of our patients are at their wits' end. Some already have consulted numerous specialists and tried multiple prescription medications—either to no avail or with intolerable side effects. Others have gone the natural route, experimenting with ginseng and other herbs to improve their mood or enhance their energy.

In fact, the number one reason most of our patients say they buy supplements is to boost flagging energy. Yet the majority of herbs and nutrients touted for their energy-enhancing properties actually offer little benefit or cause unpleasant side effects.

But *Rhodiola rosea* is different.

By now you may be wondering, How can one herb do so much? And if it really is so special, why haven't you gotten wind of it before now? The answer—which we'll discuss in much greater detail in chapter 4—is part folktale, part Cold War thriller. For centuries, *Rhodiola rosea* has been prized by those who live in the regions where it grows. It wasn't systematically studied by scientists until the latter half of the 20th century. And many of the results of those investiga-tions were kept top secret until recently.

In part 2, we will present convincing scientific proof of how

Rhodiola rosea—which thrives in unforgiving subarctic terrain—can dramatically improve nearly every aspect of our physical and mental well-being. But because this resilient herb directly increases energy in cells, we first must explore the key role of energy in our overall health.

WE ARE ENERGY

We tend to think of our bodies as solid structures—consisting of bone, muscle, organs, and a network of arteries and veins through which our blood circulates. In reality, we could condense the solid matter in the human body to the size of a thimble. The rest is space—space within cells, space between cells, space between organs. Connecting and enlivening all these parts is the energy that our cells produce. It's what keeps us going. Without an adequate energy supply, our health suffers.

The ancient Chinese healers who devised acupuncture, a healing discipline that acts directly on the body's energy centers, recognized this thousands of years ago. So did the ancient Indian scientists and spiritual teachers who created yoga techniques to elevate *prana*, the Vedic word for life force. They understood that energy is our most precious human resource. But just like the energy that heats our homes and fuels our automobiles, the energy in our bodies is finite. Our challenge is to learn to use it wisely while doing everything we can to make sure we don't run low.

Continually tapping our energy supply without replenishing it can lead to an imbalance that has a negative effect on our health and well-being. Until we learn to maintain balance between how much energy we burn and how much we store, we may be doing the best we can, but we won't be doing—or feeling—our best.

Two Tales of Energy Imbalance

Many patients who seek our help struggle to handle the multiple stresses in their lives. They have trouble just getting through the day, fulfilling their obligations, let alone experiencing moments of peace and joy. Although some show symptoms of depression, a surprising number cite low energy as their chief complaint. Without knowing anything about the science of energy, many describe themselves as feeling depleted or "running on empty." Sam and Nancy are perfect examples.

If it's Tuesday, it must be Bombay. Sam traveled so much he seldom knew where he was or what time of day it was until he opened the drapes in his hotel room. Still, he had been organizing public events for so many years that he somehow managed to pull himself together after 4 hours of sleep, then entertain an audience of 5,000 as if on autopilot. He even breezed through hours of organizational meetings in touchy political environments and situations laden with cultural sensitivities. But after 12 years of crisscrossing time zones, Sam—renowned for his incredible stamina—realized that he was running out of steam.

Sam and Dick had known each other for years. When they met by chance at a conference in Germany, Dick immediately noticed the strain in Sam's face. In the few minutes they spent together, Sam asked if Dick could help him overcome the mental and physical fatigue that was becoming his constant companion as he circled the globe.

Fortunately, Dick had a spare bottle of *Rhodiola rosea* in his backpack. He handed the bottle to Sam, who was rushing to catch a ride to the airport en route to his next destination. Two weeks later, Sam sent an e-mail of thanks praising his newfound energy booster.

Like Sam, Nancy was so accustomed to pushing herself that she didn't realize just how depleted her energy stores were. And at age 45, she was too busy and revved up to pay much attention to the changes that were taking place in her body and brain. Although she had started working part-time when her first child turned 2, after her second pregnancy, she decided to leave her job and become a stay-at-home mom. Before she knew it, Nancy was caught up in the whirlwind of raising three children. Her days were packed with the usual school functions, carpooling, and homework support, plus household chores and volunteer activities.

As her kids became more independent, Nancy decided to return to the classroom herself, to pursue a graduate degree in computer science. She signed up for two classes at a nearby state university. That's when it hit her: She was in a program with 24-year-olds who had been playing with computers since they were toddlers. Their minds processed information faster than hers. Nancy needed to spend so many extra hours on homework that she was staying up later and later. Soon she was forgetting things and losing things—signs that she was expending far more energy than she was replenishing. The demands were just too great, and the strain of keeping up with family responsibilities as well as schoolwork left her stressed and exhausted.

But Nancy was no quitter. She gave up her few leisure activities to devote more time to her studies. Then one day she felt her heart skip a few beats. Nancy's doctor explained that a combination of stress, weight gain, and lack of exercise—all by-products of her hectic lifestyle—was causing her irregular heartbeat. This served as Nancy's wake-up call. She realized that by not paying attention to her health, she had increased her risk of developing heart disease, diabetes, and cancer. She took this as a challenge, declaring to her family, "I'm not going to die prematurely from one of those age-related diseases!"

Nancy enrolled in a medically supervised weight-loss program. Every time she dropped another 5 pounds or walked an extra mile, she celebrated. But even though her weight was nearing a normal range, she still was having problems with low energy, mental slug-gishness, and forgetfulness. That's when she got in touch with Pat, who recommended *Rhodiola rosea*—100 milligrams twice a day.

A week later, Nancy called, wondering if the herb could work in just 7 days or if she was experiencing a "placebo response." She re-ported that her mind was sharper and that her memory was im-proving. Best of all, she had enough energy to carry her through the day and still enjoy the company of her husband and children in the evening. And because of all she had done to restore her health, her heart no longer skipped a beat.

For both Sam and Nancy, *Rhodiola rosea* was one of the keys to overcoming stress and fatigue. But as Nancy learned, we also must make dietary and lifestyle choices that allow our bodies to recharge and heal.

When we spend down our energy reserves without replenishing them, we shortchange ourselves. We not only fall short of our poten-tial, but we endanger our health as well. *Rhodiola rosea* can help re-plenish vital energy so we are able to make the necessary adjustments to live full, balanced lives.

CELLS: THE BODY'S POWER PLANTS

Since every action, thought, and emotion—and especially stress—uses energy, you may be wondering exactly where all that energy comes from. Each cell produces its own energy supply via the mito-chondria, microscopic structures that convert nutrients from food into energy. The cells store their energy in molecules called ATP (adenosine triphosphate) and CP (creatine phosphate), which trans-port and release energy as necessary. If our bodies were cars, ATP and CP would be the fuel in those huge storage tanks that stand near refineries, in the trucks that fill the underground tanks at the local filling station—*and* in the hose that runs from the gas pump to the car.

The instructions for producing ATP and CP are encoded in our DNA. When the mitochondria generate ample quantities of these molecules, the cells have an abundance of energy and are capable of fueling all the biological activities necessary to function optimally. But if for some reason the mitochondria can't keep up with the cells' energy demands, we're at risk for a cellular energy crisis.

Researchers have identified several factors that can impair mitochondria, thereby diminishing energy production. Among them is hypoxia, a condition in which cells don't get enough oxygen to metabolize glucose and produce ATP and CP. Hypoxia can occur at high altitudes or can result from a reduced blood supply due to atherosclerosis (hardening of the arteries), heart or lung disease, stroke, head injury, massive bleeding, or smoking. Actually, anything that inhibits the oxygen-carrying capacity of red blood cells can set the stage for hypoxia. Incidentally, *Rhodiola rosea* helps protect against hypoxic damage and has been used to prevent altitude sickness.

Another factor that can compromise the energy-producing ability of mitochondria is injury to DNA and cellular membranes. Oxygen free radicals are notorious for wreaking havoc on our bodies. But in fact these unstable molecules have the potential to do good or evil—helping to destroy infectious viruses and bacteria, or assaulting essential cellular components. The phrases *oxidative stress* and *oxidative damage* refer to the harm inflicted by oxygen free radicals on DNA and cell walls, as well as on proteins. As this damage accumulates, a cell's capacity to generate energy declines. This is considered to be a major contributor to cell death, tissue damage, and aging and age-related degenerative diseases.

Because brain cells run at a very high metabolic rate—making them the gas guzzlers of the body's energy consumers—they are especially vulnerable to oxidative damage and energy crises. When they don't have enough energy in the tank to keep running smoothly, it leads to a loss of neurons, or nerve cells. This, in turn, can accelerate brain aging and the onset of degenerative diseases such as Alzheimer's and Parkinson's.[7]

On the bright side, recent studies suggest that we can improve energy efficiency, reduce oxidative damage, and safeguard cells in the brain and central nervous system. The key is to increase our intakes of antioxidants and adaptogens such as *Rhodiola rosea*, along with making healthy changes in our diets.[4] *Rhodiola rosea* boosts energy production and defends against oxidative damage. These actions are especially beneficial in improving mental performance and preventing the deterioration of nerve cells.

THE STRESS-ENERGY EQUATION

Stress occurs whenever our activity levels exceeds our energy levels, or whenever we perceive a threat to our well-being. Ever since Hans Selye's pioneering studies in the 1930s, we've learned a great deal about stress and about the harmful effects of stress hormones on every major organ and system in the body.

Unfortunately, we haven't learned nearly as much about energy. This is because in the past researchers focused exclusively on the stress response system, without examining its impact on the energy supply. More recent investigations have shown that the stress response system regulates the body's production, delivery, and utilization of energy. And because the stress response system itself runs on energy, it, too, can fall victim to chronic energy depletion.

The two main components of the stress response system are the sympathetic branch of the autonomic nervous system and the hypothalamic-pituitary-adrenal (HPA) axis. The autonomic nervous system regulates the body's involuntary functions, including heart rate, blood pressure, the dilation and constriction of blood vessels, respiration, digestion, and the activity of smooth muscles. The two parts of the autonomic nervous system, known as the sympathetic branch and parasympathetic branch, balance each other. For example, the sympathetic branch is responsible for the release of epinephrine (adrenaline) and norepinephrine, hormones that accelerate heart rate and respiration. The parasympathetic branch has the opposite effect, slowing heart rate and respiration.

The hypothalamic-pituitary-adrenal axis regulates the manufacture and release from the adrenal gland of hormones called glucocorticoids. Among them is cortisol, which influences many aspects of homeostasis—the state of equilibrium—throughout the body, including the storage and release of fuel, suppression of the immune system, and reproduction. The sympathetic nervous system and the HPA axis use many neuroendocrine pathways to communicate and coordinate their activities.

Selye found that whenever we're subjected to excessive physical or emotional stress, the sympathetic nervous system can trigger the body's fight-or-flight response, a complex chemical reaction that helps us to handle threatening situations.[5] This remarkable "survival instinct" kicks in with the rapid release of epinephrine, norepinephrine, and cortisol—the stress hormones mentioned earlier. They stimulate our brains to be more alert while pumping more blood into our muscles and delivering the extra energy necessary to survive the immediate danger. (Actually, epinephrine and norepinephrine qualify as *neurohormones*. In other words, they act as both hormones and neurotransmitters, chemicals that enable nerve cells to communicate with each other.)

The elegantly designed stress response system is meant to be activated for relatively short periods of time, followed by longer intervals of recovery and healing. But when the crunch is ongoing and our bodies must endure prolonged high levels of stress, the epinephrine, norepinephrine, and cortisol keep on pumping. In effect, the stress hormones that are essential for our short-term survival keep our bodies running on overdrive without allowing our cells to fully replenish their energy reserves or make critical repairs.

Until quite recently, doctors and scientists believed that all we needed to do to break the stress spiral is calm the sympathetic nervous system, primarily by avoiding overexposure to stressful situations. According to the latest research, this is only half of the equation. As chapter 2 explains, the imbalance in the autonomic nervous system involves both overactivation of the sympathetic nervous system and underactivation of the parasympathetic nervous system. It is the parasympathetic branch of the autonomic nervous system that is responsible for healing and for replenishing our body's energy reserves. In order for it to do its job, we need regular intervals of recovery, during which the stress response system is not operating at warp speed.

How the Stress Response System Regulates Energy

When the stress response system switches on, the body is preparing for an emergency. Just as a race car at the starting line uses more fuel when the driver revs the engine, our bodies burn more energy when we're getting ready to fight or flee. Our brain cells are activated for increased alertness and attention to danger, so they consume more energy. So do our hearts as they beat harder, our lungs as they pump faster, and our muscles as they contract.

The body stores fuel in the form of fatty acids and glucose, a simple sugar. To meet increased energy demands during times of stress, the stress hormones mobilize energy stores by stepping up several processes, including lipolysis (the release of fatty acids into the bloodstream as triglycerides), glycogenolysis (the release of glucose into the bloodstream), and protein catabolism (the breakdown of proteins). Then the stress hormones accelerate the delivery of these raw materials by elevating heart rate, which in turn increases bloodflow to critical areas, such as the brain and muscles.

Of course, with this higher rate of consumption, energy reserves won't last very long. But once we escape from or overcome a stressor, feedback mechanisms such as cortisol switch off the stress response system, allowing the body to replenish its energy supply. Still, if the state of emergency lasts for too long, it can set the stage for an energy crisis.

ENERGY DEPLETION AND FREE RADICAL DAMAGE

Simply put, constant activation of the stress response system can deplete the body's energy supply beyond its capacity to refuel. When individual cells do not have enough energy to maintain their vital functions, different parts of the system may become fatigued, strained, and eventually damaged. This may manifest itself as chest pain or heart attack, high blood pressure, stomach irritation or ulcer, reduced immunity, or another health problem, depending on individual vulnerabilities.

In addition, when cells metabolize nutrients—which is what occurs chemically when we burn energy—they also generate by-products, including oxygen free radicals. An oxygen free radical is the molecular form of oxygen, minus a crucial electron. We're constantly burning energy and releasing oxygen free radicals, even when we eat, or talk on the telephone, or go for a walk.

Oxygen free radicals are part and parcel of being alive. But when we're under chronic or recurrent stress, we burn more energy and produce even more oxygen free radicals than usual. If the concentration of these molecules exceeds the body's capacity to neutralize them, they begin to harm cells and—in cases of chronic stress—our tissues and organs, including our brains. Oxygen free radicals also damage mitochondria, the cellular components that produce energy, thereby reducing our capacity to maintain cellular energy levels.

The overproduction of oxygen free radicals could be compared to the dumping of chemical waste. When waste products accumulate faster than the environment can detoxify them, plant and animal life suffer.

How Do We Avoid
an Energy Crisis?

Think of the parasympathetic nervous system as the Environmental Protection Agency of the body. Just as mandatory speed limits conserve fuel, the parasympathetic system reduces energy expenditure by slowing the heart and respiratory rates and calming the brain. This enables cells to slow their energy production and reduce the release of oxygen free radicals. Then the cellular defenses have a chance to neutralize any existing free radicals and repair any damage before it becomes so severe that the cells lose their capacity to produce energy and end up being destroyed.

This means that if we don't train ourselves to slow down and take time to recharge—even when the stress in our lives is positive, as with the birth of a child or a promotion at work—our energy reserves stay chronically low and we're constantly battling burnout. Even the word *burnout* is on the mark because during times of severe or chronic stress, the stress response system literally *burns* extra energy. If we remain in this state long enough without shoring up our energy supplies, our bodies become vulnerable to disease and premature aging.

The good news is, we can easily replenish the energy we use when we're under stress. How? By balancing periods of intense mental and physical activity with periods of rest; by maintaining a healthy lifestyle; and by boosting our energy reserves with *Rhodiola rosea* and other natural energizers.

Too Much Stress, Too Little Energy

Before we can stop the stress cycle, we must understand the far-ranging consequences of excessive energy depletion without adequate energy renewal—which is what occurs when the stress response system remains in high gear for long periods of time. As we noted earlier, 80 percent of all medical illnesses are triggered or worsened by stress.

Chronic overexposure to stress hormones is one of the ways in which prolonged stress can undermine our health. Over time, too-high levels of epinephrine, norepinephrine, and cortisol can lead to loss of muscle mass, decreased sensitivity to insulin (a risk factor for diabetes), high blood pressure, elevated cholesterol and triglycerides, cardiovascular disease, poor tissue repair, and suppressed immunity—not to mention impotence in men and the cessation of menstruation in women.

Of course, each of us is born with particular genetic vulnerabilities—our own weak link or Achilles' heel—that get challenged whenever we're subjected to chronic stress. Some people are more prone to heart disease, while others are vulnerable to cancer. Yet regardless of our genetic inheritance, scientists are beginning to suspect that one pivotal factor in the development of heart disease, high blood pressure, and many other illnesses is overactivation of the sympathetic nervous system and underactivation of the parasympathetic nervous system.[6]

What's more, a number of psychological conditions could point to an underlying stress/energy imbalance. For example, depression—which might be described as extreme, chronic activation of the stress response system—has reached epidemic proportions worldwide. In the United States alone, 16 percent of adults—or 35 million people—suffer from major depression severe enough to warrant treatment at some time in their lives.[2] These numbers do not account for cases of chronic low-level or subsyndromal depression, which researchers believe to be far more widespread. (We'll talk more about depression in chapter 9.)

The stress/energy imbalance can affect virtually every bodily system by manifesting itself as a host of serious health problems, including the following:

- Cardiovascular—high blood pressure, atherosclerosis, heart disease
- Neurological—impaired memory, concentration, and cognitive function; migraines and headaches; Parkinson's disease;

Alzheimer's disease and dementia; fibromyalgia; chronic fatigue syndrome

- Gastrointestinal—ulcers, irritable bowel syndrome, ulcerative colitis, Crohn's disease

- Immunological—rheumatoid arthritis and other autoimmune disorders; infections, including frequent colds, respiratory infections, and yeast infections; urinary disorders, such as frequent urges to urinate and pain upon urination; skin conditions; allergies; cancer

- Endocrine/metabolic—hypoglycemia, type 2 diabetes, menstrual irregularities, infertility, weight problems

- Musculoskeletal—muscle pain and spasms, neck and back pain, sciatica, temporomandibular joint pain

- Psychological—anxiety, panic disorder, post-traumatic stress disorder, depression, low sex drive, sexual dysfunction, sleep disorders, eating disorders, attention deficit disorder

THE STRESS-AGING CONNECTION

At the far end of the spectrum of complaints that may arise from a chronically stimulated stress response system—and the resulting stress/energy imbalance—is premature aging, along with age-related degenerative diseases such as atherosclerosis, Alzheimer's, diabetes, and osteoporosis. Despite this, centenarians now rank as the fastest-growing segment of the U.S. population.

In recent years, scientists studying longevity have advanced various theories to explain why some people live to a healthy old age and others don't. While genes may be important, the difference between longevity rates now and 100 years ago most likely stems from the significant decrease in infant mortality at one end of the age spectrum and improved geriatric care at the other end. This is especially true now that medical interventions prevent many diseases from becoming fatal. In fact, it's beginning to appear that a normal human lifespan—barring accidents and life-threatening illness—is between 100 and 120 years![3]

Although details of the complex relationship between stress and aging—involving both environmental and genetic factors—are still emerging, we have enough information to draw some basic conclusions. Not surprisingly, much of the current research suggests that an overactive stress response system seems to accelerate the aging process. According to one theory of aging known as metabolic remodeling, healthy centenarians show less damage to their cells than their less healthy peers. Metabolic remodeling is one of several theories of aging under investigation, as you'll see in chapter 4.[1]

Overall, healthy centenarians tend not to overreact to stress, and are careful to replenish their energy stores to maintain their good health. The successful adaptation of their stress response systems contributes to their longevity.

Of course, since the beginning of time, we humans have been searching for the secret to living longer. Today scientists are developing keys to unlock the human genome, as well as new tools to probe the mysteries of aging. In the meantime, we're being bombarded by a vast and confusing arsenal of "miracle" pills and potions that make outrageous antiaging claims. Some provide limited benefit, but most do nothing; most are harmless, though a few might actually be detrimental to your health.

As with most aspects of our existence, there's bad news and good news in our quest for eternal youth. The bad news is that no single potion will extend our lives forever. The good news is that we can dramatically improve our quality of life by staying as healthy as possible for as long as possible. Many people who adopt a healthy diet and lifestyle, and who do not suffer from chronic stress, are able to maintain a good quality of life up to 100 years of age—and sometimes beyond.

Sufficient energy is the sine qua non of good health. When we reviewed studies of the healthy elderly in the United States and abroad, we identified five factors as the essence of a long, productive, active life: a high-energy diet, physical and mental fitness, a strong social network, adequate sleep, and a clear, calm mind. We'll explore each one of these elements in depth in chapter 15.

In addition, because no one dwells in a stress-free utopia where life unfolds exactly according to plan, we recommend a regimen of herbal and nutritional supplements that have helped us and our patients maintain a healthy balance between energy expenditure and energy renewal. Our personal and clinical experience has taught us that an integrated approach, including the judicious use of *Rhodiola rosea* to help enhance the body's energy production, can help us live well and happily as we grapple with unprecedented demands and pressures on our time.

In other words, each and every one of us has the power to get—and stay—energized for life, even in the face of stress. *Rhodiola rosea* is vital to replenishing energy stores and maintaining that all-important stress/energy balance.

CHAPTER 2

How
STRESS
AFFECTS ENERGY

Even as *Rhodiola rosea* helps our patients recover their energy, we find that the more they grasp the science behind the stress-energy equation, the better equipped they are—psychologically and intellectually—to make the necessary adjustments to live full, balanced lives. Just as important, once they understand that an overactive stress response system depletes their energy supply, compromising their ability to function optimally, self-blame—which only fuels stress—all but disappears. They stop *should*-ing themselves—as in "I really *should* be able to work a demanding full-time job and be the perfect spouse, parent, in-law, friend, neighbor, and volunteer—plus take night classes at the community college."

The list of things that most of us are conditioned to believe we should be and do is endless, but *somethin's gotta give*. Realizing why you can't be all things to all people is the first step in learning to run on full instead of empty. It also frees you from the negative cycle of unrealistic expectations—which by definition you cannot possibly fulfill—and the consequent feelings of guilt and failure.

As Pat discovered when she was sick with Lyme disease, she needed to reevaluate everything and be very clear about what was most important for her and the people she's closest to. Because she had so little energy, anything in the nonessential category was cut back, postponed, or dropped altogether.

Taking stock of how we use our energy provides a helpful reality check. And it's absolutely essential whenever we're feeling burned-out or showing signs of physical and mental overload, such as frequent colds, low-level depression, digestive problems, or plain old irritability. We most likely are dealing with an energy deficit, brought on by unrelenting stress and a continuously stimulated stress response system.

WHAT DO WE MEAN BY STRESS?

Stress occurs whenever the demands of life exceed the ability to cope with them. A stressor can be any stimulus, external or internal, that the brain interprets as excessive or threatening. Some stressors, such as the smell of smoke, arouse a negative reaction in most people. Others cause bad feelings in one person, but good feelings in another.

For example, a person who was bitten by a dog as a child might be frightened at the sight of a canine, while someone who grew up with a family pet might feel warmly nostalgic. Similarly, skiers and mountain climbers get a rush when gazing down from a mountaintop, which probably would terrify anyone with a fear of heights.

Stressors can take many forms—environmental (heat, cold, and radiation), chemical (pesticides and pollutants, as well as oxygen free radicals and other by-products of metabolism), biological (bacteria and viruses), or psychological (a death in the family, divorce, job loss). Certainly, positive events, such as getting married or buying a new house, can be just as stressful as negative ones. Virtually anything that involves change or unfulfilled expectations can trigger a stress response. Our innermost thoughts and desires can have the same effect.

All kinds of stressors constantly bombard us. Some go away as quickly as they appear or linger for only a short time; others can recur or become chronic. Over the millennia, the human body has developed a remarkable network of defense mechanisms beyond the stress response system that enable us to adapt to a wide range of stressors.[7] These mechanisms include cellular defenses such as antioxidants, DNA repair tools, and heat shock proteins, as well as our immuno-neuroendocrine systems. Even so, any stressor has the potential to disturb our equilibrium—or homeostasis—and challenge our stress response.

How the Stress Response Works

We experience a multitude of internal and external stimuli even when we're asleep. If the control centers in the brain—which are on 24-hour alert, evaluating all those stimuli—perceive anything as cause for alarm, they activate the stress response system. As explained in chapter 1, the two main components of the stress response system are the sympathetic branch of the autonomic nervous system and the hypothalamic-pituitary-adrenal axis (HPA).

The instant the brain senses danger, whether real or imagined, the sympathetic nervous system (SNS) whips into action and mobilizes energy for fight or flight. The *locus coeruleus*—the control center of the SNS, located in the brain stem—releases norepinephrine, one of the so-called stress hormones. Norepinephrine sends messages down the spinal cord to the body's major organs, as well as up to the limbic systems and higher brain areas, and over to a part of the adrenal gland called the adrenal medulla.

The release of norepinephrine from the locus coeruleus, combined with the release of epinephrine from the adrenal medulla, increases heart rate, blood pressure, respiration, and muscle activity. It also prompts the brain to be more alert and ready for action. By narrowing some arteries and dilating others, the sympathetic nervous system diverts bloodflow to deliver more oxygen and nutrients to the body parts most in need of energy in an emergency—the heart, lungs, brain, and muscles of the arms and legs. Meanwhile, the cells use more oxygen and accelerate the release of energy by burning more glucose, a simple sugar derived from the breakdown of nutrients. This energy fuels the body's survival functions.[11, 15, 21]

Stress also activates the limbic centers of the brain—the hypothalamus, amygdala, and hippocampus. The hypothalamus produces corticotrophin-releasing factor (CRF), which activates the HPA axis and leads to the production of cortisol, another of the stress hormones. The amygdala and hippocampus play roles in emotional reactions, such as fear, anxiety, and panic, as well as in emotionally charged memories. The limbic system and the locus coeruleus use neurotransmitters and hormones as messengers, sending these substances back and forth to coordinate their activities.

Ultimately, the effects of stress depend on the intensity and duration of the stressor, as well as on a person's perception of the degree of threat. When the stressor is present only briefly, the stress response system usually copes successfully. A state of homeostasis returns quickly, thanks to the healing and recharging action of the parasympathetic branch of the autonomic nervous system.

FROM ALARM TO EXHAUSTION

The scientist Hans Selye identified three phases of an organism's stress response. The first is the alarm phase, when a stimulus triggers the body's stress response system. During this phase, activation of the SNS leads to rising levels of epinephrine and norepinephrine. These stress hormones prepare the body for impending danger, as described above. They also heighten attention and sharpen memory and problem-solving skills.[19]

Meanwhile, the HPA axis instructs the adrenal glands to increase their production of cortisol. This stress hormone mobilizes the energy supply by inducing the release of stored fat as triglycerides (lipolysis); converting stored energy to glucose (glycogenolysis); and breaking down proteins (catabolism).

If a stressor persists, the body shifts into the second phase of the stress response, known as the resistance phase. This is when cells that may have been damaged during the alarm phase are repaired and rebuilt. This process, called anabolism, also helps prepare the body for future stressors.

The third phase of the stress response, the exhaustion phase, sets in when the stressor continues beyond the body's ability to resist it. Not surprisingly, this phase is the most hazardous to our health.[19]

Prolonged, recurrent, or chronic stress can damage nerve cells, particularly in the hippocampus but also in other tissues and organs. The hippocampus is important for emotional memory and is especially vulnerable to damage by the excess levels of cortisol and neurotransmitters that can result from an extreme stressor such as childhood abuse, rape, or combat duty during war. In addition, the problem-solving skills that sharpen during the alarm phase become less and less effective during the exhaustion phase. Thinking and memory are likely to be impaired, and anxiety and depression creep in. This is especially true when a person feels unable to cope or senses a loss of control.

Most of us realize that our reactions to a perceived stressor often are out of proportion to the actual threat. In effect, we're responding to our own negative thoughts and emotions, rather than to the stressor itself. The trouble is, these negative thoughts and emotions—if they linger—can disturb the function of the autonomic nervous system and contribute to high blood pressure, heart disease, rheumatoid arthritis, and other illnesses.[10]

A multitude of psychological and social stressors can weigh on us every day. These, too, can impede cellular energy production and increase our vulnerability to illness. Some of these stressors, such as caring for an ailing parent or child, may be beyond our control. But others—taking on too many projects, running up credit card debt, making too many promises and commitments, and just plain overextending ourselves—are not. We need to get a better handle on these stressors, the ones we could do something about if only we would learn to say *No*, *Later*, or *Let me think about it.*

How we respond to stress is a deciding factor in whether or not we're able to preserve our mental and emotional energy. If we dwell on the negative and stay in the past rather than the present, we deplete these energy stores and thus undermine our capacity to lead happy, productive lives. Remember, our state of mind determines our quality of life.

A New Take on an Old Problem

In the past few years, groundbreaking research has underscored the crucial role of the parasympathetic nervous system (PNS) in healing the body from the damaging effects of stress.[9] As we noted in chapter 1, scientists long believed that the best way to counteract stress was to minimize the fight-or-flight response activated by the sympathetic nervous system. They underestimated the importance of replenishing depleted energy reserves, which is the job of the PNS.

They also misinterpreted the role of the vagus nerve, which research now shows to be *the* information superhighway of the parasympathetic system, relaying messages back and forth between the brain and the major systems of the body. When we were in medical school in the 1970s, we were taught that the vagus nerve (from the Latin *vagary*, to wander) exits the brain stem and then meanders on an irregular course, with branches that regulate the heart, lungs, and gut—but that was about it. Back then, scientists assumed the vagus was more or less a one-way street.

It now appears that only 20 percent of the vagal fibers carry information from the brain to the body, while the remaining 80 percent make the return trip—transmitting information from millions of sensors in body organs and systems to the relay control centers in the brain stem. From there, a vast complex of signals ascends to the limbic system and to widespread areas of the cerebral cortex.

Think of it this way: If the body were a symphony orchestra, the vagus nerve would be the conductor—interpreting the music, setting the tempo and volume, listening to each instrument, harmonizing the various sections of the ensemble, and influencing the emotional tenor of the work. Similarly, the vagus nerve engages in constant three-way communication between the limbic system (the seat of our emotions), the cerebral cortex (which processes our thoughts and perceptions), and the body's major organs and systems.

The vagus nerve also is a major conduit for mind-body interactions—so the next time you experience a "gut reaction," you'll know that your vagus is speaking to you. Interestingly, the vagus (sometimes called the 10th cranial nerve) even plays a role in *how* we communicate, since it affects the movements of the throat, vocal cords, neck, and face.[15]

When we experience stress, the sympathetic nervous system revs up the heart rate and instructs the body to burn more energy. But the vagus nerve, which is central to the calming action of the parasympathetic nervous system, slows the heart and conserves energy. Studies suggest that this calming action protects against stress-related damage, which can contribute to a host of health problems, including depression and cardiovascular disease.[8, 9]

HOW THE VAGUS NERVE INFLUENCES STRESS RESPONSE

The term *cardiac vagal tone* refers to just how much the vagus nerve slows the heart, based on the nerve's output, or level of activity. The higher the cardiac vagal tone, the greater the influence of the vagus nerve on the heart.

Breathing causes a normal variation in heart rate, called respiratory sinus arrhythmia (RSA). This is because with every inhalation, there is a decrease in vagal output and a corresponding slight increase in heart rate. Conversely, every exhalation elevates vagal output, leading to a slight reduction in heart rate. By using the variations in heart rate with respiration to calculate RSA, we can estimate cardiac vagal tone and vagus nerve activity. We also can measure RSA using the frequencies emitted by a beating heart. (To learn more about this technique, see the opposite page.)

Researchers have found that infants with high RSA—which indicates a high cardiac vagal tone—were better equipped to respond to the environment than infants with low RSA, who tended to be timid, fearful, or depressed.[2] Similarly, a high RSA in grade-school children predicted greater social and empathic abilities, especially in boys.[6] Perhaps most compelling, Stephen Porges, Ph.D., director of the Center for Developmental Psychobiology at the University of Illinois at Chicago, has linked certain types of vagus nerve activity to specific symptoms in autistic children. Dr. Porges is using this information to develop new treatment approaches for autism.[16]

In contrast, adolescents and adults who are aggressive or antisocial are likely to have both a low heart rate and a low RSA, which suggests underactivity of both the sympathetic and parasympathetic branches of the autonomic nervous system.[13, 14] Further, low cardiac vagal tone is associated with depression, anxiety disorders, and panic disorder.[5, 20] And among patients with coronary artery disease, those

---

New Tool Shapes New Understanding of the Vagus Nerve

Respiratory sinus arrhythmia (RSA) offers a means of measuring vagus nerve activity. But it is only one of many factors that can cause variations in heart rate. For example, both the sympathetic and parasympathetic nervous systems influence heart rate, as do body temperature, chemoreceptors, and baroreceptors—that is, nerve receptors that are sensitive to chemical stimuli or changes in pressure.

As each of these factors acts on the duration of the heartbeat cycle, it generates a particular set of frequencies. Scientists have developed a technique called heart rate variability, which can separate the different frequencies and determine their corresponding influences. One current definition of RSA is a heart rate variability in the high-frequency band, between 0.12 and 0.40 Herz.[18] This high-frequency band can accurately measure the effects of the vagus nerve on variations in heart rate—in other words, cardiac vagal tone.

The discovery that vagus nerve activity can be measured indirectly by tracking changes in heart rate and calculating heart rate variability has been a major breakthrough in vagus nerve research. Now scientists can study the role of the vagus nerve in many physical and psychological conditions without the invasive procedures once necessary.

who have an underactive parasympathetic nervous system also tend to have a poorer prognosis and survival rate.

As you can see, the activity of the parasympathetic nervous system has a significant impact on many aspects of emotional and social development, as well as on general health. The therapeutic potential of improving parasympathetic function is just beginning to be recognized.

IT'S ALL IN THE WIRING

Everyone is wired differently, with some of us having more reactive stress response systems than others. Whether it's the result of nature or nurture, or a combination of the two, that's just how we're built.

The issue of having a highly sensitive stress response system comes up all the time in our practices. Audrey, one of Pat's patients, reports that she frequently feels as though something terrible is about to happen, even though she knows better. She is exquisitely sensitive to criticism and to the facial expressions, tone of voice, and unspoken needs of everyone around her. Even though her coworkers value her because she is so tuned in to them and so careful to treat them with kindness and consideration, she still worries about being disliked. She needs a lot of "alone time" at home, after dealing with people all day at work. Bright lights and loud noises bother her, too.

Audrey and others with especially sensitive stress response systems frequently worry that they're somehow defective. What's more, they blame themselves for their sensitivity. This isn't the case for everyone, however. Those with sensitive stress response systems who are raised by supportive parents learn how to soothe themselves and how to rise to meet life's challenges. It's no coincidence that once they reach adulthood, many of these people excel in the arts, in nurturing professions, and in leadership roles.

Of course, some with sensitive stress response systems have not received what the British psychoanalyst D. W. Winnicott once described as "good enough" mothering.[22] Often these people endured early losses, separations, and traumas that kept them from learning how to repair the damage caused by a hair-trigger fight-or flight response. Perhaps more than anyone, they need to attune themselves to the delicate balance between their stress and energy levels, taking extra care to replenish their energy reserves as soon and as often as possible. With time, they may be able to overcome the stresses from early in their lives and "train" their stress response systems to not always be on high alert. Some people may need guidance from a counselor or therapist to facilitate recovery.

In her book *The Highly Sensitive Person*, Elaine Aron describes the pluses and minuses of extreme sensitivity. These people can be quite empathic, creative, and attuned to subtleties. At the same time, they may overreact to emotional, sensory, and social stimuli.[1]

It is interesting to note that while highly sensitive people tend to have overactive stress response systems, violent criminals are the polar opposite, with generally underactive stress response systems.[2, 4, 14] In fact, their brains seem to become most active when they're engaging in risky, impulsive, or aggressive behavior. In a certain sense, they're addicted to stress. The rest of the time, they feel dull and unfocused.

CHANGING THE WIRING

Although those who engage in violent activities and those who are highly sensitive are at opposite ends of the stress response spectrum, considered together they suggest one of the fundamental paradoxes of being human. Our minds crave change and stimulation, while our bodies—including our stress response systems—thrive on the familiar. On the one hand, we find comfort in our favorite foods, those well-worn sneakers, the same old rituals and routines. On the other, we are excited by new sensations, new ideas, new challenges.

And so life becomes a constant balancing act as we humans strive to offset the rush of the sympathetic nervous system with the recharging action of the parasympathetic nervous system, excitement with calm, the desire to discover new people and places with the reassuring sameness of family and home. Once we achieve a healthy balance, we may discover that opposites can be complementary.

Obviously, we have no control over a good deal of what happens in our lives. But we do have the power to choose—if only whether to spend an extra hour on the computer late at night and risk draining our last drop of energy, or to acknowledge our bodies' signals and get the sleep we need. Likewise, we can choose to limit our reliance on the extraordinary technology now available to us, which encourages near-constant stimulation of our minds and bodies—often at the expense of our health.

Perhaps most important, we can choose our reactions to life's events and surprises. By becoming more aware of our thoughts and emotions, we can catch ourselves chewing over things that have upset us or made us feel hurt, insulted, or angry. Once we realize that we're wasting valuable energy by churning up our stress response systems, we can learn to let go and return to a state of calm. In the long run, our health and vitality depend on the wisdom of our choices.

While each of us is wired in a particular way, our nervous systems have much more plasticity—or capacity for change—than we might imagine. For example, we constantly absorb new information because the nerves in our information processing and memory centers can make new connections. That's plasticity.

You may wonder why mastering a new computer program or learning a new skill is relatively easy, while altering a gut reaction is virtually impossible. The reason is that in general, changing our emotional wiring is more difficult. But it can be done, at least to some degree. In particular, corrective emotional experiences—in the form of healthy relationships, creative expression, spiritual practices, and many forms of psychotherapy—can help to liberate us from overreactive response patterns.

What's more, adjustments in diet and lifestyle, including the use of *Rhodiola rosea*, can help tone the stress response system and support the healing brought about by corrective emotional experiences. *Rhodiola rosea* takes the edge off sensitivity and anxiety, enabling people to remain calmer and cope better—whether they have normal or overreactive stress response systems. When combined with other positive changes in diet, lifestyle, and mindset, *Rhodiola rosea* is even more effective in stabilizing the stress response system and improving physical health and emotional well-being.

STRESS IS NOT A FOUR-LETTER WORD

As we learn to respect and work with the rhythms of our unique stress response systems, we need to recognize that *not all stress is all bad all the time*. After all, if we didn't react to certain stressors—food burning on the stove, an ambulance racing up the highway, a child crying after a fall—few of us would get through the day. We depend on the stress response system to protect us and those we love. It alerts us to danger, quickly boosts energy levels, and mobilizes the physical and mental defense mechanisms necessary to deal with a wide range of stressors.

What's more, a certain amount of stress helps develop our capacity to cope with the unexpected. It also increases our endurance, enabling us to accomplish personal goals—perhaps lifting weights or running a marathon.

When athletes train for competition, they place just a little more stress on their bodies each time they work out. In response, their bodies adapt to the gradually increasing demands. Experts refer to this process as *hormesis*, a term originally used to describe the effects of substances that were benign or beneficial in small amounts but toxic in large quantities.[17] This definition has been expanded to incorporate the idea that mild stress—whether physical or mental—may strengthen an organism, while severe stress may damage it.[3]

For example, most people understand that if they gradually increase the intensity or duration of their workouts—a mild form of stress—their strength and endurance will increase in turn. On the other hand, if they were to attempt a 5-mile run without first building up to it, they likely would end up with very sore muscles, if not a more serious injury.

In much the same way, mild stress may help to maintain the elasticity of the stress response system. To see a healthy stress response system in action, just watch a happy baby suddenly start to cry, then a moment later let out a belly laugh, his cheeks still wet with tears. Babies can switch from one mode to the other in the blink of an eye. That's a perfect example of the interplay between the sympathetic (reactive) and parasympathetic (recharging) branches of the autonomic nervous system.

What happens as we grow older is that we become worn down by repeated or prolonged stress. Our stress response systems lose their innate elasticity. Without realizing it, we become more rigid and less adaptable.

WAYS TO BUILD STRESS RESISTANCE

Research has shown that invigorating traditions such as the Scandinavian sauna can improve the elasticity of the stress response system. Scandinavians first take a hot sauna, then pour a bucket of ice-cold water over their heads, and finally rewarm themselves in a sauna or hot tub. The cold temperature of the ice water shifts the stress response system into high gear, causing the sympathetic nervous system to rapidly burn energy. The hot water has a soothing effect, which allows the parasympathetic nervous system to invoke calm and replenish energy stores. Taken in its entirety, the sauna sequence helps tone the whole stress response system by building resilience in the face of stress. It's kind of like a stress vaccination.

In a similar way, restricting calories—while maintaining adequate intakes of essential vitamins and minerals—creates a state of mild physical and emotional stress that may not only boost resistance to more severe stressors but also strengthen the body, reduce the risk of disease, and even extend lifespan. While the discovery that calorie restriction could prolong the lives of laboratory rodents by 30 percent occurred some 30 years ago, it only recently has become the focus of research involving humans. Now longevity studies suggest that people who ate a healthy diet of between 1,700 and 1,900 calories a day tended to resist illness and live longer.

Research at the National Institute on Aging has found that calorie restriction triggers a type of cellular stress response, stimulating cells to produce proteins called neurotrophic factors. These proteins enable neurons, or nerve cells, to grow new "arms" (axons and dendrites) that make new connections with other neurons. Neuronal plasticity—that is, the ability of neurons to make new connections— is essential for learning and adaptation.

In animal models of human neurological medical conditions such as Alzheimer's, Parkinson's, and stroke, calorie restriction protected neurons from degenerating. It also stimulated neurogenesis, or the production of new neurons—which may compensate for cell loss from aging and injury.[12] Other research has shown that calorie restriction improved cellular resistance to the damage caused by free radicals and other substances.

The bottom line is this: Exposure to mild stressors, coupled with periods of recovery, can build our energy reserves and help to restore the interplay between our sympathetic and parasympathetic nervous systems. This is essential to maintain the stress/energy balance and to reap the rewards of good health and longevity.

RHODIOLA ROSEA
WORKS BEST UNDER STRESS

Stress uses energy. When we react appropriately and consistently to the stressors in our lives, we build our resistance while maintaining our energy stores. But if a stressor overwhelms our ability to cope, it drains our energy supply and wipes out any opportunity to recharge. Left unchecked, a particularly severe or persistent stressor can damage the body's defense mechanisms, leaving us vulnerable to psychological distress as well as physical illnesses, such as heart disease and high blood pressure.

The parasympathetic nervous system is critical to regulating our stress response. *Rhodiola rosea* enhances parasympathetic function and fortifies the stress response system, improving our ability to overcome stress and reducing our risk of stress-related health problems. As you will discover in part 2, *Rhodiola rosea* actually works best in stressful situations. It's a potent antidote to today's hectic, high-anxiety world.

CHAPTER 3

Finding
YOUR OWN
STRESS/ENERGY BALANCE

How do you know if you have an overreactive stress response or depleted energy stores? The following three self-assessment tools can help. We created them exclusively for this book so you can evaluate how much stress you're experiencing, how well you maintain your energy supply, and whether your stress response system is running on overdrive.

Once you identify your personal tendencies and patterns in each of these three areas, you can begin making appropriate adjustments to restore and maintain your stress/energy balance. If you find that you have an especially sensitive stress response system, you'll need to take extra care to replenish your energy reserves. Be sure to read chapter 15, which offers strategies for creating an energizing diet and lifestyle.

Of course, *Rhodiola rosea* can play in important role in normalizing an overreactive stress response. It also can be beneficial if your stress level is high or your energy is low. Either way, it helps restore balance.

Before you take these quizzes, you may want to make photocopies of them for later. Or write in pencil so you can reuse these pages as often as you wish. That way, you can track your progress in managing stress and maximizing energy.

In each quiz, place a check mark next to each statement that applies to you most of the time, then count up the total. The key that follows each quiz will help you evaluate your score.

Quiz I: How High Is Your Stress Level?

1. ___ I get upset too easily.

2. ___ I have been irritable lately.

3. ___ I know I overreact to things.

4. ___ Calming down is hard for me.

5. ___ I don't seem to be able to relax.

6. ___ I tend to worry a lot.

7. ___ I feel tense.

8. ___ I spend too much time thinking about things that went wrong in the past.

9. ___ I focus on what's wrong and feel pessimistic.

10. ___ I am hypercritical of myself and others.

11. ___ I don't feel motivated.

12. ___ I have trouble getting things done at work or school.

13. ___ I don't get satisfaction from my job.

14. ___ My energy level is low.

15. ___ I don't get enough sleep/rest.

16. ___ I am not getting enough exercise.

17. ___ I feel tension in my neck, shoulders, or back.

18. ___ I'm having a conflict with a family member, friend, or coworker.

19. ___ I can't seem to get over a recent loss.

20. ___ I feel under pressure.

___ Count the number of checks to determine your stress level.

0–5: Low   6–10: Moderate   11–15: High   16–20: Severe

The quiz above can help zero in on the stressors in your life—the reasons that you feel irritable, worried, sad, or tired. Think of these areas as ripe for change. If your score is high and you can't figure out why, you may want to discuss it with a trusted family member or close friend, or even consult a counselor. This person may offer insights that can help pinpoint the source of your stress.

Quiz II: How Well Do You Replenish Your Energy Supply?

1. ___ I get at least 7 hours of sleep a night, on average.

2. ___ When I am doing intense work, I remember to take breaks to walk, stretch, or relax.

3. ___ I eat three balanced meals a day.

4. ___ My diet is high in protein.

5. ___ My diet includes at least three servings of fruit and three servings of vegetables a day.

6. ___ I rarely eat sweets or fatty foods.

7. ___ I eat fish on a regular basis or take supplements of omega-3 fatty acids.

8. ___ I take a good-quality multivitamin every day.

9. ___ I take antioxidants and a B-complex supplement every day.

10. ___ I usually drink at least 6 glasses of water every day.

11. ___ I engage in moderate- to high-intensity exercise at least three days a week or walk for 30 minutes at least five days a week.

12. ___ I practice meditation, yoga, yoga breathing, tai chi, or another form of relaxation.

13. ___ I have a close, loving relationship with my partner and/or family.

14. ___ I have good friends; we support one another.

15. ___ I have a strong sense of faith or engage in spiritual practices.

16. ___ I find meaning in my relationships, my job, and life in general.

17. ___ I enjoy activities that are different from my job, such as art, music, dancing, competitive sports, or gardening.

18. ___ I participate in community service activities.

19. ___ I volunteer to help others, and it's rewarding to me.

20. ___ I often go outside to enjoy nature, fresh air, and sunshine.

_____ Count the numbers of checks to assess your energy needs.

16–20: Recharging optimally
11–15: Breaking even
5–10: Running low
0–5: Running on empty

This quiz above shows you what you're doing right to boost your energy supply. It also may give you new ideas for generating energy that you haven't considered before. Improving your diet and sleep habits, getting regular exercise, and practicing relaxation techniques take time, effort, and commitment. Joining forces with a friend or a group can help achieve your goals. Remember, the higher your stress level is, the more energy you need.

Quiz III: How Sensitive Is Your Stress Response System?

1. ___ I feel pain, tension, or a knot in my stomach.

2. ___ I get tension headaches.

3. ___ I overreact when something goes wrong.

4. ___ I startle easily; sudden loud noises make me jump.

5. ___ I'm frightened by certain people or situations.

6. ___ I become paralyzed with fear.

7. ___ I get so nervous I can't speak.

8. ___ I get so angry I lose control.

9. ___ I yell and say things that I regret.

10. ___ I always need to feel in complete control.

11. ___ I don't trust people in general.

12. ___ I feel threatened.

13. ___ When I get anxious, my heart pounds or beats fast.

14. ___ I don't adjust well to change.

15. ___ I tend to imagine the worst.

16. ___ I feel overwhelmed and cannot get things done.

17. ___ I feel like I'm moving in slow motion.

18. ___ I feel hopeless.

19. ___ Sometimes life does not seem worth living.

20. ___ I tend to get sick a lot.

_____ Count the number of checks to determine the status of your stress response system.

0–2: Mildly overactivated
3–7: Moderately overactivated
8–15: Highly overactivated
16–20: Severely overactivated

If your score on the quiz above suggests that you have a moderately overactive stress response system, you probably can calm it by paying closer attention to your diet and exercise habits and to your sleep and relaxation patterns. More than likely, taking *Rhodiola rosea* and engaging in an activity like yoga or meditation will be enough to provide the daily de-stressing you need.

On the other hand, if you have a highly or severely overactive stress response system, it may be interfering with your ability to do your job or to have satisfying relationships. The three laws of energy balancing that follow, as well as the strategies in chapter 15, should help rein in your stress response. If stress persists and your energy level plummets, consider seeking professional help. Psychotherapy or counseling may be just what you need to learn how to lower your stress level and raise your energy reserves.

THE THREE LAWS OF ENERGY BALANCING

Maintaining your energy supply is a dynamic, ongoing process. We'll explore numerous ways of accomplishing this throughout the book, and especially in chapter 15. Underlying our approach are these three fundamental laws of energy balancing.

Energy Law #1: You Must Replenish Your Energy Reserves Continuously

Taking a 1- or 2-week vacation each year—even if we manage not to check voice mail and e-mail—simply cannot begin to undo the damage wrought by 50 weeks of energy overspending. Nor can slowing down for 1 day a week—a good strategy, as the keepers of the Sabbath know—compensate for a 6-day energy deficit. You need to take steps every single day to rest your stress response system and rev up your parasympathetic nervous system to replenish your energy reserves. This is because energy, like the ocean tides, ebbs and flows throughout the day.

The first step—and the bedrock of healthy energy renewal—is to get a good night's sleep. Second, incorporate periodic breaks into each day. These respites from physical and mental strain can take many forms: walking in the fresh air alone or with a friend, listening to music, shooting hoops with a coworker, meditating at your desk for 5 to 10 minutes, practicing deep breathing or tai chi, or just stretching for 5 minutes. Do whatever works best for you.

For some people, short naps do the trick. Winston Churchill, who took a nap every day, once said: "You must sleep sometime between lunch and dinner. You will accomplish more. When (World War II) started, I had to sleep during the day because that was the only way I could cope with my responsibilities."

Because food is our most direct source of energy, we cannot overemphasize the importance of healthful eating. Taking *Rhodiola rosea* is essential, too. You'll find guidelines for a high-energy diet in chapter 15, along with recommendations for our favorite energy-boosting herbal and nutritional supplements.

ENERGY LAW #2: YOUR ENERGY SUPPLY IS UNIQUE AND CONSTANTLY FLUCTUATING

Two guiding principles are at work here. First, the ebb and flow of your energy level is as individual as your thumbprint. While a coworker may seem to thrive on 5 or 6 hours of sleep a night or never need a break during the day, the same may not hold true for you. In reality, everyone requires periods of recovery to perform at a consistently high level. Just ask any athlete.

Energy Drains

Life is filled with challenges that deplete energy and exact a toll on body, mind, and spirit. Here we highlight the primary culprits in each category.

Physical: Not enough sleep; poor diet; too little exercise, or too much exercise without adequate recovery time; cigarette smoking; excessive alcohol consumption; illness; lack of attunement to the fluctuating rhythms of the body, as well as the rhythms of day and night and the changing seasons.

Mental: Overwork; too many responsibilities and commitments; excess stimulation from too many hours spent watching television or plugged in to computers, video games, cell phones, or e-mail; obsessive thinking and planning; insufficient downtime to just be in the present moment.

Emotional: Major losses or transitions; persistent negative emotions, such as anger, fear, worry, blame, guilt, and shame; denial of emotions; disconnecting from others, or giving too much to others when under stress; saying yes to anyone or anything; lack of joy and pleasurable activities.

Spiritual: No sense of meaning or purpose greater than oneself; isolation from others.

Second, even if your energy baseline remains fairly stable, your need for downtime will vary. You may go through periods when you must pay extra attention to recovery and repair—when you're under considerable stress, for example. At other times—perhaps when you're involved in an exciting new project at work or you've fallen madly in love—you may seem to have energy to spare.

This is why assessing your energy on a regular basis is so important. It will help establish an internal feedback loop that increases your awareness of your own, fluctuating energy rhythms. After a while, the process becomes automatic. You'll instinctively know how much energy you require to feel and perform your best.

With practice, you can restore the elasticity of your stress response system so you easily shift from coping with stress to rebuilding energy. The result is that you have a more even and consistent energy flow, without dipping too far into your reserves. Consequently, you have more energy to spend—and you recover faster when you spend it.

Energy Law #3: The Best Way to Build Energy Is Slowly, over Time

You can restore and maintain your energy supply even as you age. The secret is to do so gradually. This principle is well known among athletes, but it governs building endurance in virtually every endeavor—from lifting weights to writing a book. The challenge is to balance increased stress with adequate recovery time while being mindful of your individual energy rhythms.

Of course, you can't control the stressors that you encounter in daily life—just as you can't control whether your boss moves the deadline for your report from next month to 4 o'clock this afternoon, or whether another driver looks down for 1 second too long and rear-ends your car. Stress—no matter what its source—uses extra energy. The rule of thumb is this: The more severe the stress, the more depleted your energy reserves and the more pressing your need for extra recovery time. No matter what you may be dealing with, once the shock wears off, you must mobilize your innate resilience.

Energy Enhancers

You can do a great deal to replenish your energy reserves so that you can meet life's demands without becoming stressed-out and endangering your health. And it doesn't involve quitting your job, packing up your family, and moving to a mountaintop!

The sources of energy renewal that are presented throughout this book will support every aspect of your well-being. For the sake of clarity here, we have categorized them according to their primary benefits.

Physical: Regular sleep habits; healthful diet; *Rhodiola rosea* and other energy-boosting supplements; regular moderate exercise; physical activities such as dancing, cycling, sailing, or team sports; yoga, tai chi, or martial arts; yogic breathing; sexual intimacy; adjusting your schedule to accommodate fluctuating energy levels.

Mental: Meditation for a calm, clear mind; daily intervals of quiet time; creative endeavors that tap a part of your brain that doesn't get much use at work or when fulfilling family or other obligations; not wasting energy ruminating on the past or worrying excessively about the future; developing a clear vision of yourself and your values and priorities; letting go of the small stuff.

Emotional: Becoming aware of and working through negative emotions; communicating openly and honestly; pursuing pleasurable activities; allowing for "alone time"; being your most authentic self, which means speaking your own truth without blaming others.

Spiritual: Becoming active in a community whose values reflect your own—a church, synagogue, temple, or mosque, or any spiritual, religious, artistic, or political group; volunteering for a cause that you care about; practicing forgiveness toward others who may have hurt you; committing random acts of kindness.

MAKING MOLEHILLS
OUT OF MOUNTAINS

Being aware of what drains your energy and learning how best to replenish your reserves is the first step toward taking charge of your health and well-being. Unfortunately, making the necessary changes *also* uses energy, especially in the beginning. All too often people are so worn down by chronic stress that they lack the desire, the motivation, and the can-do attitude that are necessary for changing old patterns. *Rhodiola rosea* can help by jump-starting your energy, lifting your mood, and quieting your anxiety. Then you can see that those mountainous obstacles to change are nothing more than molehills. That's when you're ready to begin down the path to a less stressed, more energized existence.

The discovery of *Rhodiola rosea*'s ability to enhance mental and physical performance under stress may be among the most intriguing sagas in herbal medicine. In part 2, we will share more of this herb's fascinating history. In addition, we will present cases studies from our clinical practices of patients who have experienced *Rhodiola rosea*'s remarkably wide-ranging benefits. (We've changed names and other identifying information to safeguard our patients' privacy.) Perhaps you're dealing with one or more of the health problems that we address. If so, you may want to talk with your doctor about adding *Rhodiola rosea* to your self-care regimen.

PART II

What
RHODIOLA
ROSEA
CAN DO
FOR YOU

CHAPTER 4

Why Is
THIS HERB
DIFFERENT?

For the past quarter-century or so, the airwaves have been abuzz with news of the latest herbal supplement that will improve our health and, possibly, extend our lives. We've heard about *Gingko biloba*, kava kava, ginseng, St. John's wort, and numerous other popular herbs. Why the tidal wave of interest?

The number-one reason that people turn to alternative treatments like herbs is that conventional treatments have failed to make them well. What's more, the public is increasingly aware that an ounce of prevention is vastly preferable to the disruptive, costly, and often painful interventions that are necessary to fight disease once it gains a foothold. Add to this the unwanted side effects associated with many prescription drugs, and you can see why the time is right for herbs and other "natural" therapies.

A Brief but Fascinating History

So where does *Rhodiola rosea* fit into the picture? Although this plucky herb remains relatively unknown in the West, in folk medicine it has a legendary history dating back thousands of years. We know, for example, that the ancient Greeks used *Rhodiola rosea*. In 77 A.D., the Greek physician Dioscorides documented the medical applications of the plant, which he then called *rodia riza*,[15] in his classic medical text *De Materia Medica*.[37]

But how did *Rhodiola rosea* travel more than 2,000 miles from the remote Caucasus Mountains, where it grows wild, to ancient Greece? Our search for the answer to this question took us back more than 3,000 years, to the 13th century B.C.—the Greek Bronze Age. That's when trading expeditions crossed the Aegean Sea, the Hellespont (Dardanelles), the Sea of Marmara, the Bosphorus, and the Black Sea to a land called Colchis,[38] in what is now the Republic of Georgia.

One of the best-known myths of this era celebrates the voyage of Jason and his famous crew, the Argonauts, which included Hercules and Orpheus. Like most myths, the story of Jason, the Argonauts, and the Golden Fleece blends fact with fantasy. But it hints at an intriguing theory of how *Rhodiola rosea* might have made the incredible journey to Greece from its native land.

The Greeks were not the only ancient people who valued *Rhodiola rosea*. The Vikings depended on the herb to enhance their physical strength and endurance, while Chinese emperors sent expeditions to Siberia to bring back "the golden root" for medicinal preparations.[23] The people of central Asia considered a tea brewed from *Rhodiola rosea* to be the most effective treatment for cold and flu. Mongolian physicians prescribed it for tuberculosis and cancer.

In Siberia to this day, it is said that people who drink *Rhodiola rosea* tea will live to be more than 100. The herb still is given to newlyweds to assure fertility and the birth of healthy children. For centuries the details of how and where to harvest the wild root were a closely guarded secret among members of certain Siberian families, who would transport *Rhodiola rosea* down ancient trails in the Altai and Caucasus mountains and trade it for Georgian wine, fruit, and honey.[14, 28]

In 1725, the Swedish botanist Carl Linnaeus gave the herb its modern name, *Rhodiola rosea*, and recommended it as a treatment for hernia, hysteria, headache, and vaginal discharge.[21, 22] Fifty years later, it earned a place in the first Swedish pharmacopoeia,[27] a complete listing of all medicinal preparations.

THE PLANT THAT CAME IN FROM THE COLD

Studies of *Rhodiola rosea* currently are under way in Russia, the Republic of Georgia, Bulgaria, the United States, Sweden, Norway, Japan, and China, among other countries. But much of the existing research was conducted by Soviet scientists during the Cold War, with the findings concealed in classified documents. While some of the early studies were available to the public, they were published in Slavic languages not read by Western scientists.

Research on *Rhodiola rosea* and other medicinal herbs was part of the Soviet Union's great push to compete with the West in military development, the arms race, space exploration, Olympic sports, science, medicine, and industry. During World War II, the Soviet government drafted scientists to work on projects for the military, with a focus on physical and mental performance. The Soviets were determined to find substances that would help their soldiers overcome combat fatigue and win on the battlefield.

(continued on page 56)

Rhodiola rosea's Fantastic Voyage

The myth of Jason, the Argonauts, and the Golden Fleece was passed down from generation to generation by oral tradition, and kept alive in epic poems—among them one written in the 1st century A.D. by the Roman poet Gaius Vallerius Flaccus.[39] The oldest surviving version of the story is attributed to Apollonius of Rhodes, a Greek poet who lived in the 3rd century B.C.[2, 12, 40]

As Apollonius tells the tale, Jason's uncle Pelius ruled Greece. To prevent his nephew from taking power—as was his due—Pelius sent him on a dangerous voyage to find the Golden Fleece,[41] secretly hoping that Jason would never return. Having survived many perils, Jason sailed his ship, the *Argo*, across the Black Sea toward Colchis:

> And lo as they sped on, a deep gulf of sea was opened, and lo, the steep crags of the Caucasus Mountains rose up, where with his limbs bound upon the hard rocks by galling fetters of bronze, Prometheus fed with his liver an eagle that ever rushed back to its prey.[42]

Prometheus the Titan had provoked the wrath of Zeus by giving knowledge of fire to mankind. As punishment, Zeus ordered him to be chained to a rock for 30,000 years. Every day a "Kaukasian" eagle devoured his liver, and every night his liver grew back. Each time the eagle returned to its nest, the gore from the Titan's liver dripped from its beak onto the high mountain crags.

When the Argonauts reached Colchis, Jason asked the king, Aetes, to give him the Golden Fleece. Of course, the king was loath to part with his treasure, so he demanded that Jason first prove himself worthy by subduing two fire-breathing bulls and using them to plow and plant a field with dragon's teeth.

The king's maiden daughter, Medea—a master herbalist and sorceress—had fallen deeply in love with Jason, under a spell cast by Eros and Aphrodite. She knew that even if her beloved survived the bulls, he would be slaughtered by an army of soldiers that would sprout from the dragon's teeth.[43] She appealed to her patroness, the goddess Hecate,[44] for a potion that would save Jason. Hecate showed Medea where to find an herb that would make Jason invincible. According to Flaccus, the Roman poet:

It sprang up new-formed when the flesh-tearing eagle caused bloody ichor from the suffering Prometheus, to drip to the ground on the Caucasian crags. Its flower rises on twin stalks a cubit [18 inches] high. In color it resembles the Korykian crocus [saffron], and the root in the earth is like newly cut flesh. Like the dark moisture from an oak on the mountains, she [Medea] had gathered its sap[45] in a Caspian shell . . . [46]

Apollonius's description of the plant that Medea used to create the Charm of Prometheus conforms in every detail with the herb that we now call *Rhodiola rosea*. No other plant growing in the Caucasus Mountains comes even close to a match.

After brewing her potion, Medea sped in her chariot to a secret meeting with Jason. She gave him the charm, warning him that it would last for only one day. According to Apollonius:

Then Jason sprinkled the drug all over himself: a mighty force entered him, inexpressible, without fear, and his two arms moved freely as they swelled with bursting strength . . . [47]

With his indomitable strength, Jason defeated the bulls and the soldiers. Still Aetes refused to part with the Golden Fleece. Although tormented about deceiving her family, Medea helped Jason steal her father's treasure. Together they escaped and fled to Greece, marrying en route.

Upon their arrival in Greece, Medea used her deadly potions to protect Jason from his enemies. But Jason was unfaithful and chose another bride. Euripides wrote a play in which Medea, driven mad by Jason's betrayal, sought revenge and killed their children. Other versions say that she took their children to a distant land, where she was revered by a people called the Medes.

For 2,000 years, scholars have pored over the texts of Greek epic poems. Poets and healers have searched for clues to the identity of the mysterious Charm of Prometheus. No one ever guessed that the source of the charm was none other than the ancient herb *Rhodiola rosea*.[48]

Studies involving Soviet soldiers found that amphetamines and other chemical stimulants were indeed effective for improving performance—but only in the short term. When taken for prolonged periods, they became harmful and addictive. The search continued for other substances that could increase energy and endurance without the insidious side effects.

Dr. Nikolai Lazarev was a member of the team of researchers assigned to this task. He was especially intrigued by a group of herbs that were considered "elite" or "kingly" in ancient healing disciplines. In traditional Chinese medicine, for example, these herbs were known to increase physical and mental endurance, reduce fatigue, improve resistance to disease, and enhance longevity.

Despite thousands of years of use by inhabitants of China, Korea, Japan, Siberia, Russia, and parts of Europe, these herbs had never been scrutinized in the lab. So in 1948, Dr. Lazarev and his protégé, Dr. Israel Brekhman, set out to study the chemical composition and biological activities of these herbs. Would they live up to the legend surrounding them?

A SPECIAL CLASS OF HERBS

Dr. Lazarev and Dr. Brekhman, along with a team of researchers from the Siberian Academy of Sciences, tested 158 herbal folk remedies from the Soviet Union, Europe, and Asia. They determined that some of the remedies contained extracts from plants with exceptional abilities to promote what they described as "a state of nonspecific increased resistance." In other words, certain herbs support the healthy function of every system in the body and protect it from biological, chemical, environmental, and psychological stressors.

Dr. Lazarev coined the term *adaptogen*, from the Latin *adaptare*, to describe this special class of herbs.[11, 20] Further, he and his team of scientists established three fundamental criteria that identify an herb as an adaptogen:

- Nonspecific resistance—the herb must increase the body's resistance to a broad range of agents, including physical (heat, cold, and exertion), chemical (toxins and heavy metals), and biological (bacteria and viruses).

- Normalizing action—the herb should normalize whatever pathological changes or reactions have occurred. For example, regardless of whether the thyroid gland is under- or overactive, a true adaptogen will help steer it toward normal function.

- Innocuous effects—the herb must cause minimal, if any, physiological disturbance or side effects and be very low in toxicity.

After identifying the properties of adaptogens, the Soviet researchers set about developing a test to screen for them. Studies found that adaptogens increased the amount of time that rats actively swam in a beaker of water. Later, a French scientist named Porsolt modified this test by adding some specifications to it. For the past 40 years, researchers have used the Porsolt swim test to screen substances for antidepressant activity.

The development of this test led to rigorous studies to confirm which of the widely heralded herbs in fact help the body *adapt* to all sorts of unfavorable conditions, from combat, space travel, and Olympic competition to everyday stress. In 1968, Dr. Brekhman published the results of these studies. Of all the herbs selected for testing, only four met the criteria of a true adaptogen: *Eleutherococcus senticosus* (sometimes called Siberian ginseng or eleuthero); *Panax ginseng* (Asian ginseng or Korean ginseng); *Rhaponticum carthamoides* (rhaponticum or luzea); and *Rhodiola rosea* (golden root, roseroot, or Arctic root). Subsequent research added *Schizandra chinesis* (schizandra) and *Withania somnifera* (ashwagandha) to the list.[8]

Since 1968, scientists have learned much more about the properties of adaptogens, leading to the expansion of the original definition to encompass the new information.[11] According to the updated definition, a true adaptogen also must help modulate the body's stress response system so that it reacts in proportion to actual danger, instead of overreacting and depleting cells of vital energy. This is especially important under conditions of extreme stress, such as sustained physical exertion, toxic exposure, and mental or emotional strain.

What's more, a true adaptogen must demonstrate a balancing effect on the body's regulatory systems, including the cardiovascular, immune, and neuroendocrine systems.[25]

HOW ADAPTOGENS HELP

More than 50 years of research have firmly established the positive influence of *Rhodiola rosea* and other adaptogens on the central nervous system. In 1987, Soviet scientists Al'bert Samoilavich Saratikov and Efim Abramovich Krasnov published the results of dozens of experiments showing that *Rhodiola rosea* enhanced cognition, perception, concentration, learning, and memory.[29] Subsequent research has confirmed these findings.[4, 32]

Adaptogens such as *Rhodiola rosea* also improve the body's immune defenses by increasing the production and activity of specialized cells—including natural killer cells and T cells—that fight bacteria, viruses, and cancer. And thanks to their multiple benefits, from enhanced energy production to antioxidant activity and DNA protection, these "wonder herbs" may reinforce the body's ability to resist mutagenesis, the process by which healthy cells turn cancerous.

On the stress front, research has shown that adaptogens guard against the release of excessive amounts of stress hormones, notably cortisol, epinephrine, and norepinephrine. This is important because too much of the stress hormones for too long can cause unnecessary wear and tear on the body. What's more, when taken over time, adaptogens appear to enhance the flexibility of the stress response system, enabling it to protect the body against a wider range of stressors.

As we learned in chapter 2, the stress response progresses through three phases: alarm, resistance, and exhaustion. Adaptogens can help during all three phases. In fact, much of the research on adaptogens has concentrated on their ability to reduce the body's stress response during the alarm phase. And by increasing stress resistance, these herbs effectively delay the onset of the exhaustion phase. A good analogy is talking on your cell phone while it's plugged in: You're consuming energy and recharging your battery at the same time. In much the same way, adaptogens boost energy while you burn energy, helping to maintain your reserves and avert burnout.

Although scientists have yet to advance a single theory that accounts for the diverse benefits of adaptogens, studies point to several important mechanisms that make these medicinal plants frontline defenders against the effects of stress. First of all, they improve cellular energy production by raising levels of the essential high-energy molecules ATP (adenosine triphosphate) and CP (creatine phosphate)—both critical players in maintaining our energy reserves. Second, because they are powerful antioxidants, adaptogens protect mitochondria (the cellular components responsible for generating energy), cell membranes, and DNA.[30] Third, they help maintain the healthy function of cells and organs by increasing the manufacture of proteins and other substances necessary for repair. And fourth, these potent jack-of-all-trades herbs protect against damage by improving cellular efficiency, reducing oxygen consumption, enhancing cardiovascular function, and reinforcing the elasticity of the autonomic nervous system.[2, 18, 31]

Of all the herbs used throughout the world and studied by scientists, adaptogens are the most effective in reducing stress and preventing many of its harmful consequences. And they have the fewest side effects.

NOT YOUR TYPICAL STIMULANTS

As we mentioned earlier, Soviet scientists tested numerous stimulants—including amphetamines—during World War II in an effort to identify those that would reduce fatigue and increase endurance in soldiers. The benefits of these substances are fleeting because they rapidly deplete epinephrine and norepinephrine. So, after the initial rush, they cause energy levels to plummet, setting the stage for exhaustion, addiction, and mental instability. Fortunately, the search for substances that could boost energy and endurance *without* the harmful side effects led to the discovery of adaptogens.

The availability of these herbs is welcome news for people who are trying to juggle the often competing pressures of their professional and personal lives—especially now that the use of illegal stimulants, notably methamphetamine (also known as speed, ice, and crystal), has reached epidemic proportions. Tragically, a significant number of those relying on illegal stimulants are working women overwhelmed by the challenges of balancing family and career. On college campuses, many students turn to stimulants when studying for exams, only to end up "crashing" or becoming addicted. People from all walks of life are paying a terribly high price for too much stress on the road to success.

Everyday stimulants, such as caffeine, nicotine, and chocolate, are no great shakes either. Like many of their illegal counterparts, they provide an instant power surge, followed by a precipitous drop in energy. Used repeatedly, they also can cause addiction, not to mention jitteriness, irritability, headaches, and other unpleasant side effects.

By comparison, adaptogens offer a more moderate energy boost— one that does not exhaust the system and that allows for rapid recovery from stress. Just as important, their benefits accumulate over time, without the risk of addiction or unwelcome side effects.

In fact, just as measured increases in exercise gradually build flexibility and strength, the regular use of adaptogens gradually improves the body's ability to respond in an appropriate manner to stress, instead of automatically kicking into high gear as though even relatively minor or moderate stresses were catastrophes. And as noted before, adaptogens make the autonomic nervous system more flexible, so it can handle a broader range of stressors and quickly return to a state of equilibrium once a stressor goes away. In other words, adaptogens can safeguard energy reserves at the same time they're fine-tuning the stress response system.

RHODIOLA ROSEA VERSUS OTHER ADAPTOGENS

So how does *Rhodiola rosea* compare with other adaptogens and medicinal plants? Since only a few studies have focused on the similarities and differences among medicinal herbs, the best we can do to answer this question is evaluate the quantity and quality of the research, then add our own clinical experience into the mix. We should point out that some herbs—notably *Eleutherococcus senticosus*, *Panax ginseng*, and *Rhodiola rosea*—have been the subjects of extensive investigation, while others have been largely ignored. The absence of solid scientific research leaves a question mark regarding their value in healing, even though they may be quite useful.

As you read about all the adaptogens and compare their benefits (refer to the charts beginning on page 76), you will understand why *Rhodiola rosea* has become our favorite. Ever since the "golden root" helped Pat recover from Lyme disease, we've had many opportunities to validate the scientific research in our clinical practices. We've seen patients who take *Rhodiola rosea* get better and better, both physically and psychologically. And they don't suffer the troubling side effects caused by many prescription drugs and, in some cases, by other adaptogens.

We also have recommended *Rhodiola rosea* in combination with a variety of prescription medications, as well as other herbs. In some cases, it has increased the effectiveness of the companion treatments; in other cases, it has minimized their unpleasant side effects. Regardless of its specific action, *Rhodiola rosea* time and again has improved our patients' health and vitality, as well as their outlook on life.

In the following chapters, we'll explore how *Rhodiola rosea*—sometimes in combination with medications or other herbs—can enhance mental and physical health, especially when people are under stress. Better than any other substance we know of, this hardy herb works both sides of the stress-energy equation, calming a sensitive sympathetic nervous system and stimulating a sluggish parasympathetic nervous system. In this way, it helps restore balance to body and mind.

THE JEWEL IN THE CROWN
OF ADAPTOGENS

Rhodiola rosea grows wild in the high, dry, rocky mountain ranges of northern Asia, Mongolia, and Siberia, as well as in the subarctic regions of Alaska, Europe, and Scandinavia. If you were to hike about 10,000 feet into the Altai mountains of Siberia in summer, when the passes are clear, you might spot a swath of yellow *Rhodiola rosea* flowers blooming on the cliffs just below the snow line. The fact that the plant can thrive in such harsh conditions—cold, wind, drought, reduced oxygen, and intense radiation exposure—might explain its exceptional healing power.

Rhodiola rosea has a tough, pale root containing a dark sap. When cut, the root gives off the aroma of a rose—hence the species name *rosea*. From the root, tough stems rise 12 to 30 inches. Sometimes multiple stems sprout from the same root. Blooming at the top of each stem is the striking yellow flower.

In extensive animal and human testing, *Rhodiola rosea* has proven to be a model adaptogen. It not only enhances performance, it also aids survival against the most severe physical stressors—from extreme heat or cold, to toxic chemicals (including chemotherapy drugs), to cancer. What's more, it helps the mind and body overcome psychological stressors, such as sleep deprivation, depression, and post-traumatic stress disorder. Perhaps most significantly, it could increase longevity by reducing the damage associated with age and illness. (For an overview of some current theories on aging and their respective links to *Rhodiola rosea*, see page 64.)

Like other adaptogens, *Rhodiola rosea* has very few side effects. It is extremely safe and nontoxic. From studies involving animals, scientists have determined that the herb would be unlikely to cause serious physical harm in humans unless the dose exceeded 20,000 milligrams. Considering that the usual clinical doses range from 100 to 400 milligrams a day, the margin of safety is enormous.[19, 34] In fact, *Rhodiola rosea* is safer and has less toxicity than most of the prescription and over-the-counter remedies that people use every day.

How We Age

Researchers have developed many theories to help explain the complexities of the aging process. This table presents the prevailing schools of thought. In the right-hand column, you can see how the actions of *Rhodiola rosea* might complement each one.

WHAT THE THEORY MEANS	HOW *RHODIOLA ROSEA* MIGHT WORK
Network Theory Cellular defenses form an interconnected system that enables cells to deal with diverse physical, chemical, and biological stressors. When these defenses fail, cell senescence (cell aging) can set in.	*Rhodiola rosea* may delay cell aging by bolstering cellular defenses that overcome diverse physical, chemical, and biological stressors.
Membrane Theory Over time, damage to cell membranes (walls) by free radicals exceeds the cells' capacity for repair. This leads to loss of membrane fluidity and impairment of cellular functioning, contributing to the processes that cause illness and aging.	*Rhodiola rosea* helps to prevent free radical damage to cell membranes.
Remodeling Theory Healthy centenarians are better able to adapt to damaging stressors by successfully "rewiring," or remodeling, their stress response systems. Their stress responses are neither too strong nor too weak, but just right.	*Rhodiola rosea* helps to balance and improve the function of the stress response system. This contributes to successful remodeling.

WHAT THE THEORY MEANS	HOW *RHODIOLA ROSEA* MIGHT WORK
Metabolic Remodeling Theory Insulin resistance occurs when the hormone insulin becomes less effective in helping cells utilize glucose. As a result, fat stores increase and blood sugar rises, generating oxygen free radicals and other forms of tissue damage. This can contribute to coronary artery disease.	*Rhodiola rosea* reduces insulin resistance, counteracts excess fat storage, and protects against oxidative damage.
Inflamm-aging Excessive inflammatory response, coupled with genetic vulnerabilities, can lead to age-related diseases such as atherosclerosis, diabetes, osteoporosis, and Alzheimer's.	*Rhodiola rosea* reduces inflammation, as shown by diminished C-reactive protein and creatine kinase.[1]

THE PHYTOCHEMISTRY OF
RHODIOLA ROSEA

Identifying the active compounds in adaptogens such as *Rhodiola rosea* has been challenging, to say the least. For one thing, there are so many active compounds. For another, as scientists attempt to sort out which of the known chemicals are responsible for the various healing actions, they keep discovering new ones.

Here's what we know so far. The root of the *Rhodiola rosea* plant contains these six groups of bioactive compounds.

- Phenylpropanoids: rosavin, rosin, rosarin
- Phenylethanol derivatives: salidroside (rhodioloside), tyrosol
- Flavonoids: rhodiolin, rodionin, rodiosin, acetylrodalgin, tricin
- Monoterpines: rosiridol, rosaridin
- Triterpines: daucosterol, beta-sitosterol
- Phenolic acids: chlorogenic acid and hydroxycinnamic acid, gallic acids

By the 1980s, *Rhodiola rosea* was in such demand in the Soviet Union that it became overharvested.[9] With supplies dwindling, some companies began substituting other plants in products touted as rhodiola. The loss of therapeutic effect in a number of popular preparations prompted an investigation by the Soviet government. Scientists discovered that salidroside, the compound that they had been using as a chemical marker for *Rhodiola rosea*, was present in many other plants. Unscrupulous companies could easily substitute worthless herbs containing enough salidroside to pass quality testing.

This finding sparked a search for other compounds that were unique to *Rhodiola rosea* so scientists could accurately identify and standardize products claiming to be the *real* herb. As a result of their efforts, they found three unique phenylpropanoids that exist only in *Rhodiola rosea*: rosavin, rosin, and rosarin. The term *rosavins* refers to all three.

The 1989 Soviet pharmacopoeia set forth the new standard that products sold as *Rhodiola rosea* must contain 3 percent rosavins and 0.8 to 1.0 percent salidrosides. This replicates the ratio found naturally in the roots.[24] In order to provide maximum health benefits, products should contain rosavins and salidrosides in a 3:1 ratio.

RHODIOLA ROSEA
FOR MAXIMUM EFFECTIVENESS

If you decide to try *Rhodiola rosea*, be absolutely sure to buy a high-quality brand of pure root extract that contains a minimum of 3 percent rosavins and 0.8 to 1.0 percent salidrosides, as mentioned above. If the product label does not list the respective percentages of rosavins and salidrosides, contact the manufacturer. If the manufacturer is unwilling to provide this information, then look for another brand.

The label also should say that the product contains only *Rhodiola rosea*, not a mix of *Rhodiola* species. If the label says just "rhodiola" or "arctic root," you have no way of knowing if it is the right species.

Refer to page 229 of the resource section for a list of some reliable supplement brands. Avoid Internet bargains and products without adequate evidence of quality control.

ALCOHOL OR WATER EXTRACT?

Traditionally, people prepared *Rhodiola rosea* root as a tea, by extracting the herb in hot water. Today manufacturers extract the herb using hot water, alcohol, or sometimes both. While any of these

Not All *Rhodiola* Plants Are Created Equal

By now you may have noticed that we never refer to our favorite adaptogen by only its first name: *Rhodiola*. We do this for a very important reason. We want to be sure that if you decide to try this herb, you take *Rhodiola rosea* and not another *Rhodiola* species.

Scientists have identified 16 other species within the *Rhodiola* genus. Though some have shown promising adaptogenic properties in animal studies, very few have undergone testing in humans. On the other hand, the number and quality of animal and human studies involving *Rhodiola rosea* offer compelling evidence to support the therapeutic value and safety of the herb. That's why, until more research is done on other members of the *Rhodiola* genus, we're not comfortable recommending them.

methods yields a bioactive product, there probably are some differences in their phytochemical compositions.

LIQUID, TABLET, OR CAPSULE?

In the Soviet Union, people buy *Rhodiola rosea* as a concentrated root extract in a small amount of alcohol. It also is available as a liquid tincture, with the dosage measured in drops. As of now, we can't purchase the herb in either liquid form in the United States.

Here root extracts of *Rhodiola rosea* are available as tablets or capsules. The tablets tend to come in higher doses. We prefer the capsules because they allow for more flexibility in dosing. Also, those who may be sensitive to the herb can open a capsule and remove a smaller amount, which they can mix into juice or tea.

Before buying a *Rhodiola rosea* product, read the label to determine the amount of herb in each tablet or capsule. A single capsule, for example, generally contains between 100 and 200 milligrams.

For simplicity, we've based our recommended dosages of *Rhodiola rosea* on 100-milligram capsules. If you buy a product that supplies

170 milligrams per capsule, remember to adjust your maximum dosage to two capsules (340 milligrams) or possibly three capsules (510 milligrams) a day, as opposed to four of the 100-milligram capsules.

Storage and Use

Tablets and capsules made with *Rhodiola rosea* root extract are stable and so do not require refrigeration. Although the herb can be paired with food, it is much better absorbed on an empty stomach. We recommend timing each dosage 20 to 30 minutes before a meal or 2 hours after.

Since *Rhodiola rosea* is stimulating, it is best taken first thing in the morning and at midday, ideally before breakfast and lunch. It should not be taken in the late afternoon or evening because it may disrupt sleep.

In the following chapters, we will provide dosage information that we've tailored to specific health concerns. In general, as with any medicinal substance, your best bet is to start with a small dose of *Rhodiola rosea*—for example, one 100-milligram capsule 30 minutes before breakfast—and observe how your system responds. If you notice no effect after 3 days, then add another capsule 30 minutes before lunch. Once you feel more energetic or you see some improvement in your mood, mental alertness, memory, or physical endurance, stay at the same dose for at least 3 weeks to determine how much benefit you get. If you think that you need a slightly bigger boost, add a third capsule before breakfast, then wait another 3 to 7 days before—if necessary—adding a fourth capsule before lunch.

The average dose of *Rhodiola rosea* is 200 to 400 milligrams a day. Some people respond to as little as 25 milligrams a day, while others may need as much as 600 or even 800 milligrams, depending on the nature of their problem, their physical size, and other factors. If you think that you need more than 400 milligrams a day, we suggest that you seek the guidance of a physician who is familiar with the use of the herb.

Although *Rhodiola rosea* has a high safety profile and low toxicity, it has yet to be systematically tested in doses exceeding 400 milligrams a day. For this reason, we strongly advise against taking more than 400 milligrams a day without medical supervision. We have seen at least one product that supplies 1,000 milligrams of *Rhodiola rosea* per capsule. To date, there is no evidence to suggest that such high doses provide any additional benefits. And they could cause adverse effects, unless future research proves otherwise.

If you forget a dose of *Rhodiola rosea* before mealtime, you can take it during or after your meal without problem. The only downside is that it may not be absorbed as well. If you miss a dose completely, simply resume taking the herb according to schedule the next morning, rather than try to catch up at dinner or later. It could interfere with your sleep then.

SIDE EFFECTS

Some people are sensitive to the stimulating effects of *Rhodiola rosea*; they say that they feel agitated, jittery, or "wired" when taking the herb. If this happens to you and you also are consuming caffeine, try cutting back on coffee, black tea, and caffeinated soft drinks. If overstimulation continues to be a problem, you may need to temporarily decrease your dosage of *Rhodiola rosea* and build your tolerance more gradually. You can do this by taking just a fraction of a capsule and then increasing your dosage by one-half capsule every 2 weeks.

If you experience intense dreams once you begin taking *Rhodiola rosea*, don't worry. They should subside in about 2 weeks. If you're troubled by a little nausea, try taking two ginger capsules 20 minutes before your dose of *Rhodiola rosea*, or drinking a cup of ginger tea.

MEDICAL PRECAUTIONS AND DRUG INTERACTIONS

If you have a medical condition, it always is wise to check with your doctor before trying any herbal product. If your doctor is not familiar with *Rhodiola rosea*, give him a copy of this book or suggest reading our phytomedicinal review of the herb in the November 2002 issue of *HerbalGram* magazine.

We do advise caution for anyone with bipolar disorder (manic depression) who is prone to agitation or manic episodes. This is because any treatment that increases energy, like *Rhodiola rosea*, also has the potential to induce mania in people who are bipolar. Those who fall into this category should try the herb only under the close supervision of a doctor—and then only when their mood swings (particularly manic or hypomanic episodes) are well controlled by a mood stabilizer.

Rhodiola rosea has not shown any adverse interactions with prescription medications or with other herbal products. Be aware, though, that if you are taking a stimulating medication, *Rhodiola rosea* may increase the stimulant action.

To date, no controlled scientific studies have examined the effects of *Rhodiola rosea* in women who are pregnant or breastfeeding. There is no reason to think that the herb would be harmful, but until we have more information, we do not feel comfortable recommending it for moms-to-be or new moms.

A BRIEF TOUR OF LANDMARK ADAPTOGENS

While *Rhodiola rosea* is our adaptogen of choice, it is one of a handful of true adaptogens that have shown promising health benefits. We hope that the following overview of the rest of these herbs will help you get a handle on the properties—as well as the advantages and disadvantages—of each one.

PANAX GINSENG

The word *ginseng* comes from the Chinese *gin* (man) and *seng* (essence). Translated, it means "the crystallization of the essence of the earth in the form of man."[12]

Panax ginseng grows wild in the mountains of Asia. Its medicinal properties were first documented in the *Sen-nung Pen ts'ao-ching,* the most ancient Chinese pharmacopoeia. In fact, *Panax ginseng* had so many health benefits that it was considered the gold standard of adaptogens long before scientists began studying *Rhodiola rosea.* This led to other herbs with strong medicinal effects being called ginsengs, regardless of their species. To add to the confusion, the real *Panax ginseng* has been marketed under many names, including Asian ginseng, Korean ginseng, Japanese ginseng, and white ginseng.

Dozens of animal studies have shown that *Panax ginseng* enhances stress resistance, as well as physical and mental performance.[35] A review of 34 human studies found that most participants—from athletes and students to the elderly—experienced similar improvements.[10] While a few more recent studies did not support the earlier findings,[16] they also did not use uniform standards to test the herb. All things considered, the weight of evidence still favors *Panax ginseng* as a beneficial adaptogen worthy of further research.

In the human studies, the side effects of the herb were infrequent and mild—though we must point out that this outcome is common in clinical research involving healthy subjects. As with any other herb or drug, the use of *Panax ginseng* by the general public may bring to light additional side effects.

Moreover, long-term use of the herb—especially in doses exceeding 3 grams a day—is cause for concern. Some adolescent boys and others who have taken megadoses of *Panax ginseng* to build strength and endurance have experienced estrogen-like effects, such as painful swelling of the breasts. Other adverse reactions also have been reported, usually with larger doses. These include high blood pressure, insomnia, skin eruptions, diarrhea, irritability, agitation, confusion, and depression.

Because all but one of the studies involving *Panax ginseng* ran for 3 months or less, we don't have good data on its long-term effects. The herb is considered unsafe for children and should not be taken by women who are pregnant or breastfeeding.

ELEUTHEROCOCCUS SENTICOSUS

By the 1950s, wild *Panax ginseng* had become scarce and expensive, so Soviet scientists began studying other plants with similar properties. Among them was *Eleutherococcus senticosus*, which caught the researchers' attention because of its long history of use as a strength builder in the folk medicine of Russia and other parts of Asia.

Like *Panax ginseng*, *Eleutherococcus senticosus*—a thorny shrub that grows in Siberia and northern China—has many aliases. It commonly goes by the name eleuthero, but it also is known as Asian ginseng, Oriental ginseng, Siberian ginseng, and Russian ginseng. The herb's only real connection to true ginseng is its family of origin: Aralaceae.

Though extensive animal and human studies have shown that eleuthero has all the adaptogen effects of *Panax ginseng*, testing of some preparations failed to confirm the results.[16] This may have occurred because of the use of less potent products or because of differences in test design. In any event, the replication of earlier studies with more modern techniques would provide valuable information.

Eleuthero is remarkably low in side effects. Rarely, it can cause headaches, insomnia, diarrhea, slight increases in blood pressure, and rapid or irregular heartbeat. It is not recommended for women who are pregnant or breastfeeding, or those who have hormone-sensitive cancers. Eleuthero can trigger mania in bipolar (manic-depressive) patients or agitation in schizophrenics.

RHAPONTICUM CARTHAMOIDES

Rhaponticum carthamoides—rhaponticum or luzea for short—grows wild in the high mountains and forests of southern Siberia and Kazakhstan. It also has been cultivated in Bulgaria and Russia for use as a strengthening tonic.

Animal studies have shown that rhaponticum mildly stimulates the central nervous system, improves memory and learning, and increases work capacity—all with very low toxicity.[26] Reportedly, it also helps in cases of impotence, as well as depression or anxiety—most notably those with "hypochondriac syndrome." Be aware that these benefits are drawn from clinical observations, not controlled studies.

More recent animal studies suggest that rhaponticum not only has antibacterial and anticancer effects, it also stimulates production of red blood cells.[5, 17, 33] More clinical trials are necessary to identify possible side effects and establish guidelines for safe use.

SCHIZANDRA CHINENSIS

Although *Schizandra chinensis* has not undergone the extensive study of other adaptogens, Soviet scientists considered it an important ingredient in their sports performance formulas. The herb, which grows in China (hence its names Bei Wu Wei Zi and Chosen-Gomischi), has a long history of use in Chinese medicines.

Like other adaptogens, schizandra improves concentration and endurance and has anti-inflammatory, antidepressant, and calming actions, as well. Preliminary research suggests that it may protect the body against HIV (human immunodeficiency virus).[16] In animal studies, it reduced the effects of stress on mood, cognitive function, glucose tolerance, immune defenses, and sexual function.[7] Active ingredients extracted from the fruit of the herb may improve liver function and protect against liver damage.

Schizandra's potential side effects include heartburn, acid indigestion, stomach pain, and allergic skin reactions. Its safety during pregnancy and breastfeeding has not been established.

WITHANIA SOMNIFERA

Withania somnifera, better known as ashwagandha, is a traditional Ayurvedic medicine. In India, where its use dates back more than 2,500 years, it is considered a *rasayana*—the term for herbs that increase resistance and longevity and improve general health and well-being.[36] In other words, ashwagandha appears to be an adaptogen.

Studies show that the herb indeed provides many of the same benefits as other adaptogens, including stress reduction, memory enhancement, enhanced immune function, and antioxidant activity.[6] Ashwagandha occasionally causes stomach upset and, more rarely, skin rashes. It is not recommended for use during pregnancy or while breastfeeding.

The True Adaptogens at a Glance

Here you can see and compare the six true adaptogens in terms of their actions, benefits, and uses. For reference, ↑ indicates an increase.

ADAPTOGEN	PHYSIOLOGICAL ACTIONS	BENEFITS AND USES
Panax ginseng (Asian ginseng, Korean ginseng)	↑ Nitric oxide in immune cells, blood vessels, and erectile tissues ↑ Adrenocorticotrophic hormone (ACTH) and cortisol ↑ Protein synthesis	Antistress Antifatigue Muscle strength and recovery time Reaction time and alertness Intellectual performance Immune function and cancer prevention Sexual function Most beneficial for people over 40
Eleutherococcus senticosus (eleuthero, Siberian ginseng)	↑ ACTH and cortisol ↑ Norepinephrine ↑ Serotonin ↑ Protein synthesis	Antistress Strength and endurance Intellectual productivity Immune cell response Resilience during cancer treatment
Rhodiola rosea (golden root, roseroot, arctic root)	↑ Cellular energy production ↑ Protein synthesis ↑ Serotonin, norepinephrine, and dopamine Supports DNA repair Antioxidant, anticarcinogenic, anticancer Improves oxygen utilization	Antistress Antifatigue Anti-arrhythmic Antibiotic Energy, physical and mental performance Strength, recovery time, work capacity Alertness, memory, accuracy, learning ability Sexual function Depression, anxiety, post-traumatic stress disorder Menopausal symptoms Fibromyalgia, chronic fatigue syndrome Parkinson's, stroke, traumatic brain injury Altitude sickness Liver detoxification and protection Side effects of chemotherapy

ADAPTOGEN	PHYSIOLOGICAL ACTIONS	BENEFITS AND USES
Rhaponticum carthamoides (luzea)	Stimulant Immune stimulation ↑ Protein synthesis	Antistress Antibiotic Strength, endurance, work capacity Liver health Fatigue, weakness after illness Giardiasis
Schizandra chinensis (schizandra)	Anti-inflammatory Antioxidant Improves oxygen utilization	Antistress Antianxiety Energy, sleep, memory Physical strength and endurance Liver detoxification and health
Withania somnifera (ashwagandha)	Anabolic (builds muscle) Immune stimulation Anticancer	Antistress Physical strength and endurance

Sources: Breckhman 1968; Bucci 2000; Ernst 2001; *Natural Medicines Comprehensive Database* 2002; Wagner 1994.

Using Adaptogens Safely

By definition, true adaptogens should have few if any side effects and should have low toxicity. But like any medication, they can cause problems if you don't use them properly. Here's

ADAPTOGEN	SIDE EFFECTS
Panax ginseng	Insomnia Diarrhea Vaginal bleeding, swollen breasts ↑ Libido Headache, nervousness, vomiting with excessive use May be toxic in doses exceeding 3 grams per day—may raise blood pressure and cause agitation, confusion, depression May affect bleeding time and coagulation
Eleutherococcus senticosus	Diarrhea Dizziness Hypertension, rapid or irregular heartbeat Insomnia Headache
Rhodiola rosea	Agitation or anxiety (occasional) Intense dreams Headaches (rare)
Rhaponticum carthamoides	Overstimulation
Schizandra chinensis	Heartburn, acid indigestion, stomach pain Allergic rashes
Withania somnifera	Mild gastrointestinal upset Immune suppression

what you need to know. For your reference, ↑ indicates an increase, while ? means the information is unknown or unavailable.

INTERACTIONS	PRECAUTIONS AND CONTRAINDICATIONS
MAOI (monoamine oxidase inhibitor) drugs Anticoagulants Steroids	High blood pressure, heart disease, diabetes Bipolar disorder (manic depression)—may cause mania Discontinue 7 days prior to surgery Do not use for more than 3 months; may have long-term hormonal effects Do not use during pregnancy or when breastfeeding Do not use with steroids Not for children under age 12
Anticoagulants Interferes with some tests of digoxin levels	High blood pressure Heart disease—use with caution Bipolar disorder (manic depression)—can cause mania Schizophrenia—can cause agitation Women with hormone-sensitive cancers or conditions ? Pregnancy, breastfeeding Not for children under age 12 Lack of safety evidence beyond 6 weeks
↑ Effects of other stimulants	Bipolar disorder (manic depression)—use with caution and only when condition is under good control with mood stabilizers ? Pregnancy, breastfeeding
None known	? Pregnancy, breastfeeding
None known	Stomach ulcers, acid reflux ? Pregnancy, breastfeeding
↑ Effects of sedatives and anti-anxiety medications	Stomach ulcers Immune disorders ? Pregnancy, breastfeeding

Sources: Ang Lee 2001; Ernst 2001; Natural Medicines Comprehensive Database 2002; Wagner 1994

Rating the True Adaptogens

Can the adaptogens really do all that they claim? We've developed a rating system to evaluate the available evidence, taking into account the number and quality of scientific studies, the degree of beneficial effects, and our own clinical experience. Here's what the individual ratings mean:

++++   Substantial scientific research showing strong effects; extensive use in folk medicine; positive clinical observation of strong effects

+++   Smaller number of good-quality studies showing more moderate effects; use in folk medicine; positive clinical observations of moderate effects

++   Limited number of studies of mixed quality; use in folk medicine; positive clinical observations

	ANTISTRESS	PHYSICAL PERFORMANCE	MENTAL PERFORMANCE
Panax ginseng	+++	++	++
Eleutherococcus senticosus	++++	++	++
Rhodiola rosea	++++	++++	++++
Rhaponticum carthamoides	+	+	+
Schizandra chinensis	++	++	++
Withania somnifera	+	+	+

+	Either no scientific studies or studies that are difficult to interpret because of poor quality; use in folk medicine; some positive clinical observations
—	Lack of scientific research or inaccessible scientific research (e.g., foreign-language publication only); use in folk medicine; no clinical observations

Anabolic (ATP and CP)	Antioxidant	Immune Modulation	Anticancer
++	++	+	++
+++	++	++	++
+++	+++	++	++
++	+	++	+
++	—	—	—
—	—	+	—

Adaptogens of the Future?

The seven herbs presented here have not undergone extensive enough study to determine whether they are true adaptogens. Nevertheless, they do show some adaptogenic properties. As scientists conduct more research, some or all of these herbs may earn adaptogen

Herb	Actions
Aralia mandshurica	Antioxidant Protects against radiation
Codonopsis pilosula (dangshen)	Antioxidant Antistress Stimulant Protects against radiation Improves immune defenses
Cordyceps sinensis (cordyceps)	Antistress Improves immune defenses
Echinacea purpurea	Antioxidant Improves immune defenses
Ginkgo biloba	Antioxidant Modulates neurotransmitters May inhibit clotting by platelets
Lepidium meyenii (maca)	Aphrodisiac Energy
Rhododendron caucasicum	Antioxidant Blocks carcinogen absorption and 20% of fat absorption through intestines ↑ Energy in heart muscle ↑ Uric acid excretion Relaxes blood vessels, ↓ blood pressure

status. For your reference, ↑ indicates an increase, and ↓ a decrease. A ? means the information is unknown or unavailable.

USES	CONTRAINDICATIONS
Physical performance	Pregnancy, breastfeeding
Fatigue Diarrhea Endurance Stress tolerance	? Pregnancy, breastfeeding Needs more study

Enhances physical strength
  and endurance
Pneumonia
Respiratory infections
	May affect levels of certain medications, including
	  erythromycin, ketoconazole, carbamazepine,
	  azithromycin, antibiotics, and birth control pills
	? Pregnancy, breastfeeding

Infections	May interfere with the liver's metabolism of medications May trigger allergic reactions, asthma Stop prior to surgery ? Pregnancy, breastfeeding
Mental function Stroke prevention Erectile function Vascular disease Macular degeneration	May cause bleeding, bruising Stop 36 hours before surgery Do not use during pregnancy or while breastfeeding
Fertility Perimenopause Sexual function Malnutrition	Breast cancer, prostate cancer—do not use Occasional overstimulation ? Pregnancy, breastfeeding
Physical performance High blood pressure prevention Cancer prevention Weight loss Antigout	None known ? Pregnancy, breastfeeding

Sources: Breckhman 1968; Bucci 2000; Ernst 2001; *Natural Medicines Comprehensive Database* 2002; Wagner 1994; Zheng 2000

CHAPTER 5

REJUVENATE

YOUR MIND

Have you noticed that your memory is not quite as reliable as it once was? You might find some comfort in knowing that you're not alone and you're not imagining things. Most adults lose 1 to 2 percent of their memory capacity every year.[7]

This phenomenon—known in medical circles as age-associated memory impairment (AAMI)—has no connection to a specific disease or condition. Nevertheless, it affects nearly 6 percent of the total population and 18.5 percent of people over age 50.[2] This number climbs even higher with advancing years, as about 40 percent of those between ages 60 and 78 show signs of AAMI.[16]

While memory loss may be more common in older people, age is only one of many causal factors. Most of us, even teenagers, become more forgetful when we're tired or stressed. The picture gets more complicated when we consider that nearly everything—including our genes, environment, diet, lifestyle, health status, and even the medications we take—affects how well our brains work from infancy to old age.

Of course, we can't change our genes (at least not yet), nor can we completely eliminate exposure to environmental toxins. But we can do something about many of the other factors that influence brain function.

THE BASICS OF BRAIN HEALTH

As we mentioned in chapter 1, brain cells are high-maintenance gas-guzzlers. Like a car racing at 100 miles an hour, the brain runs at a high metabolic rate, burning a lot of fuel and releasing oxygen free radicals in the process.[18] Without adequate repair and refueling, brain cells are particularly susceptible to free radical damage. Excess free radical damage can destroy cells and accelerate brain aging, putting people at risk for degenerative diseases such as Alzheimer's and Parkinson's.[8, 28]

Making sure to get enough sleep tops the list of things that we can do to support brain cell repair. Keeping stress within an acceptable limit also is essential for mental clarity and healthy brain function. This is because brain cells, and nerve cells in general, are especially vulnerable to the adverse effects of stress.

During times of stress, nerve cells—or neurons—are bombarded with excitatory neurotransmitters and large amounts of the hormone cortisol. In response, the neurons release neurotransmitters that can either stimulate (excitatory) or inhibit (inhibitory) other neurons. In situations of extreme stress or trauma, very high levels of excitatory neurotransmitters such as glutamate can damage nerve cells, destroying delicate nerve endings and possibly causing cell death.

For example, in MRI studies, severely abused children, sexually abused women, and soldiers with post-traumatic stress disorder showed a loss of nerve cells in the hippocampus. This is believed to result from the high levels of excitatory neurotransmitters and cortisol that get released during extreme stress.[3, 4, 5]

Although a limited period of moderate stress can stimulate the mind for brainstorming and problem solving, prolonged or severe stress depletes cellular energy reserves. Over time, we begin to feel as though we're stuck in mental molasses, going nowhere fast.

Eating healthfully is another critical ingredient for maintaining healthy brain cells and brain function. Recent research has shown that we may be able to improve energy efficiency, reduce free radical damage, and prevent cellular degeneration by making dietary changes and taking nutritional supplements—especially antioxidants.[23]

Not surprisingly, bad habits can wreak havoc on brain health. Drinking too much alcohol or smoking cigarettes or marijuana—not to mention using *any* amount of cocaine, methamphetamine, or another hard drug—is toxic to brain cells. And these effects increase over time. This is because as we get older, our bodies are less able to detoxify alcohol and other substances, and our brain cells have less capacity to repair damage and bounce back to normal.

The good news is, a number of herbs, antioxidants, vitamins, minerals, and nootropics (substances that restore and maintain brain cells) have the potential to prevent, delay, and—in many cases—reverse damage to neurons. Chief among them is *Rhodiola rosea*.

THE GIFT OF *RHODIOLA ROSEA*

Cathy, a 45-year-old high school history teacher, told Pat that she was having trouble finding the right words during her lectures. Getting stuck in mid-sentence in front of her classes was embarrassing. She worried even more about losing her job or being diagnosed with early-onset Alzheimer's.

Pat suggested that Cathy give *Rhodiola rosea* a try. Soon after she started taking the herb, she reported, "My memory is so much better than it was. And now I'm never at a loss for words."

Rhodiola rosea supports brain health in a number of ways. First, at the cellular level, the herb acts as an antioxidant, reducing damage to cell membranes and those vital energy-producing cellular structures called mitochondria. Furthermore, by increasing the manufacture of the high-powered molecules creatine phosphate (CP) and adenosine triphosphate (ATP), *Rhodiola rosea* keeps these energy transporters delivering their payload wherever necessary so cells run at peak efficiency. This helps to counteract fatigue and to sustain intellectual function, especially during long hours of stressful mental work.

At the neurochemical level, *Rhodiola rosea* stimulates the production of neurotransmitters such as serotonin, norepinephrine, and dopamine, which are necessary for optimal brain function.[19, 20, 27] We know, for example, that serotonin and norepinephrine are necessary for the intellectual functions of the cerebral cortex. In addition, serotonin and other neurotransmitters affect mood and help modulate the limbic (emotional) center of the brain. As for dopamine, a decline in the level of this neurotransmitter is an unmistakable feature of Parkinson's.

Among *Rhodiola rosea*'s other brain benefits is the fact that it switches on a network of nerves in the brainstem called the reticular activating system, which literally wakes up the brain, and further increases levels of neurotransmitters. The herb also helps to balance the stress response system, preventing the excessive release of stress hormones such as cortisol, which can damage brain cells. And by improving overall physical and cardiovascular health, *Rhodiola rosea* helps the body supply the oxygen and vital nutrients necessary for the brain to run smoothly.

SOVIET RESEARCH ON MENTAL PERFORMANCE

During the Cold War, the Soviet government competed with the United States in a number of arenas, including military development, scientific achievement, and the race to conquer space. The Soviet Ministry of Defense actively sought ways to boost the productivity of its scientists and the ability of its cosmonauts to perform difficult mental tasks during spaceflight and long work shifts. In numerous mental performance tests, Soviet researchers determined that *Rhodiola rosea* not only enhanced learning and memory, it also increased mental speed and accuracy.[6, 17, 21] Further, the herb improved intellectual work capacity, abstract thinking, and reaction time. And in tests repeated over long periods, it reduced the rate of errors compared with a placebo.[22]

Although they didn't go looking for it, the researchers found that *Rhodiola rosea* had a unique dual effect: It calmed the emotions *while* stimulating the intellect. They attributed this benefit in part to the herb's ability to raise levels of certain neurotransmitters—notably serotonin, norepinephrine, and dopamine—in the brainstem, cerebral cortex, and hypothalamus.[19, 20, 27]

By the 1990s, the Soviet Union had initiated joint research projects with the Swedish Herbal Institute (SHI) to test adaptogen formulas. The goal was to find the best combination of adaptogens to enhance mental and physical performance under stressful conditions. The Soviet-Swedish collaboration produced a formula called ADAPT, also known as MPPA—short for mono- and polyphenolic acids. The formula contained three adaptogens:

- 3 milligrams salidrosides (6 to 9 milligrams rosavins) from 50 milligrams of root extract of *Rhodiola rosea*
- 3 milligrams total glycosides from 100 milligrams of extract of *Eleutherococcus senticosus*
- 4 milligrams total schizandrines from 150 milligrams of fruit extract of *Schizandra chinensis*

Extensive research confirmed that ADAPT significantly enhances energy, concentration, perception, accuracy, and reaction time.[1] More recent studies have shown that *Rhodiola rosea* alone can boost mental performance.[26]

THIS HERB STANDS ALONE

In a series of double-blind, placebo-controlled trials, *Rhodiola rosea* prevented mental fatigue, enhanced learning, reduced errors, and improved the quality of work in participants.[9, 26] Here are summaries of several of these studies, along with their respective findings.

- Among a group of 60 Indian medical students attending school in Russia, those who took 100 milligrams a day of *Rhodiola rosea* extract SHR-5 reported less mental fatigue, better physical fitness and coordination, and a greater sense of well-being than those who didn't take the herb.[25] They also performed better on their final exams, earning higher grades. (SHR-5 is a standardized *Rhodiola rosea* extract used for research purposes by the Swedish Herbal Institute.)

- Of 60 foreign students enrolled in Russian high schools, 20 received 660 milligrams a day of Rodaxin, a *Rhodiola rosea* preparation with vitamin C. Another 20 took a placebo, while the remaining 20 took nothing. The students given Rodaxin had less mental fatigue and anxiety. They also showed better work performance, coordination, and well-being.[26]

- Researchers tested the ability of 60 foreign students to learn Russian. Twenty of the students began taking 660 milligrams a day of Rodaxin, while another 20 took a placebo, and the rest took nothing. Those given Rodaxin showed a 60.7 percent increase in their language-learning ability and reported less fatigue than those not given the supplement. They also earned higher grades on their final exams.[26]

- In one especially well-documented study by the Russian Ministry of Health, in cooperation with the Swedish Herbal Institute, researchers evaluated the effects of two different doses

The Best Research Around

In medical and scientific circles, the double-blind, placebo-controlled study reigns as the gold standard of clinical research. It's much more exacting than other types of study, which means its findings are more reliable and less vulnerable to challenge.

In a placebo-controlled study, scientists randomly assign participants to take either a pill containing the active compound under investigation or a placebo—that is, a pill with none of the active compound. Nevertheless, the placebo must look, smell, and taste exactly like the real thing. This helps prevent bias in the participants' response.

In any clinical trial, a certain number of people will experience what's known as a placebo effect. In other words, they get better simply because they believe that they are taking an effective medicine. So, to accurately evaluate the benefit of a given treatment, scientists must eliminate the placebo effect by giving an actual placebo to some percentage of the study participants. Then, for example, if 25 percent of those taking the placebo and 75 percent of those taking the active compound reported improvement, we know that the compound actually would help about 50 percent of people who tried it. But if 25 percent of those taking the placebo *and* 25 percent of those taking the active compound improved, the study has not shown a therapeutic effect.

In cases where a study participant knows whether he is taking an active compound or a placebo, it could influence his response and invalidate the results. Likewise, if scientists know which participant has been given which treatment, it could sway their assessments of the responses. The term *double-blind* means that neither the participants nor the scientists know who is getting a placebo and who is getting the real thing.

Because it eliminates many potential biases, a study that's double-blind and placebo-controlled carries more weight than one that isn't. Unfortunately, implementing this sort of study is difficult, particularly when testing substances that may cause side effects. For example, if the study participants develop side effects, they may surmise that they're taking the active compound.

of standardized *Rhodiola rosea* extract on mental function in the presence of stress and fatigue. In this randomized, double-blind, placebo-controlled study, *Rhodiola rosea* showed a pronounced antifatigue action in the participants—a group of healthy military cadets between ages 19 and 21.[24] (Because findings from older scientific research are commonly criticized and dismissed, we've chosen to present a more in-depth examination of the researchers' methods and findings on page 92.)

HOW *RHODIOLA ROSEA* PROTECTS THE BRAIN

We have seen that *Rhodiola rosea* can enhance memory, attention, concentration, learning, and general intellectual performance. It also may reverse—or even prevent—the long-term effects of aging, trauma, and illness on the brain. We've noticed in our own patients that the herb helps relieve some symptoms of age-associated memory impairment, as well as Parkinson's, Alzheimer's, and attention deficit disorder (ADD). In some cases it is effective alone, while in others it works best when it is combined with medication or other herbs.

Even when there's no underlying illness, *Rhodiola rosea* can be of great benefit. As Leslie, the daughter of one of our patients, says, "My elderly father was becoming very forgetful. Although the doctors said they could not find anything medically wrong with him, I was really concerned about his driving and living alone. Once he started taking *Rhodiola rosea*, I noticed improvement in just a few weeks. Now that he's eating better and remembering things more clearly, I don't worry about him all the time."

Keep in mind that the cases we present in this chapter draw upon our own clinical observations and our colleagues'. Such anecdotal material does not carry as much weight as controlled scientific research. We hope that by bringing attention to the potential benefits of *Rhodiola rosea*, we might prompt more rigorous studies to confirm and expand upon our clinical experience.

The Brain and *Rhodiola rosea*: A Closer Look

The objective of a study conducted by Russian scientist V. A. Shevtsov and colleagues was to assess the antistress and stimulant effects of a single dose of SHR-5 *Rhodiola rosea* extract in a uniform population of healthy young men under conditions of stress and fatigue. The researchers recruited 181 cadets at the Military Institute of the Russian Federation Ministry of Defense—all on night duty, with routine military service tasks—and assigned them to one of four groups, each with specific instructions:

- Group #1 took two 185-milligram capsules of SHR-5 extract (370 milligrams of *Rhodiola rosea*).
- Group #2 took three 185-milligram capsules of SHR-5 extract (555 milligrams of *Rhodiola rosea*).
- Group #3 took two placebo capsules.
- Group #4 took no capsules.

To compare the cadets' mental performance at the beginning of the study and again over 24 hours of active duty, the researchers developed a measure that they called the antifatigue index, or AFI. It's a composite of performances on tests of speed and quality of mental task performance, short-term memory, attention, and flexibility of attention. An AFI of greater than 1.0 meant reduced fatigue and increased performance, while an AFI of less than 1.0 meant increased fatigue and decreased performance.

According to the test results, *Rhodiola rosea* bestowed pronounced antifatigue effects, as shown by the mean (average) AFI values of the four groups.

PARKINSON'S DISEASE

Neurodegenerative diseases, such as Parkinson's and Alzheimer's, involve the gradual breakdown of the central nervous system. Parkinson's affects approximately a half million Americans. In this progressively debilitating disease, damage to nerve cells leads to tremors, difficulty moving, loss of facial expression, depression, and dementia, among other symptoms. Many people with Parkinson's become withdrawn and inactive. This is what happened to Andrew, a retired sculptor, in the 11 years after his diagnosis.

- Group #1 (370 milligrams of *Rhodiola rosea*) = 1.0385
- Group #2 (555 milligrams of *Rhodiola rosea*) = 1.0195
- Group #3 (placebo) = 0.9046
- Group #4 = 0.8852

Although the differences in AFI values may appear small, they are significant because they represent a composite of many test scores. In particular, the differences between the AFIs above 1.0 and those below 1.0 are very significant, as indicated by a $p < 0.001$—in other words, the odds of getting the same results by random chance would be less than 1 in 1,000.

Beyond enhanced mental performance, the cadets who took *Rhodiola rosea* showed impressive improvement in their pulse rates and blood pressure readings. Their overall sense of well-being rose as well, as indicated by the following responses to a self-assessment questionnaire:

Group	% Feeling better	% No change	% Feeling worse
#1 (370 mg *R. rosea*)	53.7	39.0	7.3
#2 (555 mg *R. rosea*)	45.0	40.0	15.0
#3 (placebo)	17.5	70.0	12.5
#4 (control)	5.0	70.0	25.0

Shevtsov and his colleagues reported their findings in "A Randomized Trial of the Effects on the Capacity for Mental Work of Two Different Doses of SHR-5 *Rhodiola rosea* Extract versus Placebo and Control," an article published in the journal *Phytomedicine* 10 (2003), 95–105.

For more than a decade, Andrew had been rooted to an old club chair, unable to initiate any activity or conversation, seemingly lost in a confused mental state. His wife, a physician, kept searching for new treatments. Eventually, she contacted Dick. He recommended that Andrew try 400 milligrams daily of *Rhodiola rosea*.

After 1 week on the herb, Andrew got up out of his chair and went out to the garden to pull weeds. Soon he began work on a new piece of sculpture. A few weeks later, he accepted a dinner invitation from friends and actively joined in the conversation. Best of all, he was able to spend time on his own, without constant supervision.

When Dick added galanthus—an herb derived from the snowdrop plant (*Galanthus nivalis*)—to Andrew's regimen, Andrew showed even greater improvement. His coordination was so much better that he could tie his own shoelaces, which he hadn't been able to do in years. Andrew's wife described his turnaround as "a miracle," and she suggested calling Michael J. Fox to tell him about *Rhodiola rosea*.

Regardless of Parkinson's cause—which may be age, genetics, environmental toxins, cerebrovascular disease, or a history of infection[8]—*Rhodiola rosea*'s ability to boost energy at the cellular level is the most likely explanation for the herb's success in helping Andrew and other Parkinson's patients. Its benefits also may derive from its role in raising levels of dopamine and other neurotransmitters. Or *Rhodiola rosea* may inhibit COMT (catechol-O-methyltransferase) in much the same way as the prescription medication Comtan. Further research will help clarify whether one or more of these actions contribute to the herb's therapeutic value for Parkinson's.

Rhodiola rosea has made a remarkable difference in quality of life for Nathan, a successful 79-year-old businessman who developed Parkinson's after a series of strokes. Barely able to walk and terrified of falling, Nathan hadn't been doing much of anything for himself. He had become completely dependent on his wife. Making matters worse, his medication had been causing him to sleep all day and stay awake all night.

Once Nathan started taking 200 milligrams a day of *Rhodiola rosea*, his energy, mobility, and nighttime sleep improved dramatically. The addition of galantamine—a synthetic form of galanthus—further enhanced his memory and cognitive abilities. Before long, Nathan became more assertive with his wife. At first she felt nonplussed by his independent spirit, as she had grown accustomed to bossing him around. But soon she became deeply thankful that her husband was back to his old, feisty self.

ALZHEIMER'S DISEASE

Alzheimer's affects about 15 million people worldwide. In the United States, doctors diagnose about 360,000 new cases each year, and that number is rising.[12] Roughly 47 percent of Americans develop the disease after age 85, though about 3 percent get it by age 65. Those who inherit genetic forms have a higher incidence and sometimes an earlier onset, before age 60.

The devastation wreaked by Alzheimer's on the lives of people touched by it—patients, families, caregivers—is incalculable. Right now, a few treatments can slow the progression of the disease and improve mental function and daily activities for a time. But nothing can cure or reverse it.

Because Alzheimer's creates an enormous social and economic burden, scientists are looking for ways to prevent it. Studies have shown that high dietary intakes of antioxidants such as vitamin C and vitamin E may lower Alzheimer's risk.[11] Since the disease is associated with oxidative stress (damage caused by oxygen free radicals), impaired glucose metabolism, and reduced cellular energy,[14] the notion that *Rhodiola rosea* may be of some benefit makes sense.

Just like Katherine Hepburn's character in *On Golden Pond*, Mary found herself caring for her husband, Jim, after he developed dementia at age 60. Unlike Henry Fonda's character in the movie, however, Jim had a variant of Alzheimer's that comes on at a tragically early age. He had been given antioxidants and *Ginkgo biloba*, as well as many standard medications. But nothing stopped the progression of his illness.

By the time Mary brought Jim to see Dick, he was unable to finish sentences and was constantly drifting off to sleep. He was so disoriented that he required 24-hour supervision.

Dick treated Jim with a special formula called Clear Mind, which contains a blend of *Rhodiola rosea*, hydroxycinnamic acid from blueberries, and *Rhododendron caucasicum*. Although it didn't reverse his dementia, it did make him less sleepy, more alert and energetic, and better able to initiate activities and follow conversations. When Dick added galantamine to his treatment regimen, Jim's language skills returned somewhat.

Mary was grateful for these unexpected improvements. For the first time in over a year, her husband was able to attend social gatherings. The most important was a special retirement dinner, where Jim was able to recognize his old colleagues and grasp the fact that he was the guest of honor.

HEAD TRAUMA AND STROKE

In Russian studies, *Rhodiola rosea* helped patients recover from brain injury due to head trauma, as well as from vascular lesions due to ischemia or stroke—especially in the early postinjury stages.[22] (The term *ischemia* refers to a loss of blood supply to any tissues in the body—for example, the heart or the brain. If brain cells are deprived of their blood supply for too long, stroke can occur.)

Rhodiola rosea appears particularly helpful to patients with cognitive problems when combined with piracetam, a drug that increases the fluidity of nerve cell membranes and activates brain waves.[13, 29] In one large study, piracetam alone—administered within 7 hours of stroke—improved bloodflow to the areas of the brain responsible for speech[15] and enhanced language recovery.[10] The addition of *Rhodiola rosea* and *Panax ginseng* produced even better results.

Dick has used *Rhodiola rosea* to treat two women whose lives were shattered in a split second by traumatic brain injury.

Cheryl, an attractive 40-year-old divorcée, was a successful graphic designer until the day she suffered a concussion in a mountain biking accident. After her injury, Cheryl's short-term memory was so impaired that she could no longer do her job. Her career wasn't the only casualty: Cheryl's social life fell apart because she was unable to recognize social cues or control her impulses to make inappropriate comments and interrupt others. Because of her behavior, she was asked to leave the health club where she had been a member for 10 years. Her mood fell from giddy heights to suicidal depths faster than a roller coaster—a common occurrence in cases of brain trauma.

Two years after her injury, Cheryl made an appointment with Dick. She already was taking SAM-e, St. John's wort, and *Ginkgo biloba*. Dick added *Rhodiola rosea* to her existing regimen, which quickly calmed her down. Soon after, she was back at work, creating more complex designs with fewer mistakes than she had been able to since her accident. Two months later, she reported feeling "fantastic."

Now that Cheryl has added galanthus to her regimen, she's getting even better results. On her own, she has found ways to compensate for residual short-term memory loss. She has reestablished her strong social network, too.

Thirty-eight-year-old Angela, once a successful investment broker, didn't realize the seriousness of her head trauma until 10 days after she was thrown from her horse. That's when she began making mistakes at work and errors in her speech, a condition known as aphasia. A short time later, she developed difficulty concentrating and double vision. Eventually, she was diagnosed with neural fatigue, a syndrome that includes exhaustion, daytime napping, depression, and irritability.

Angela wanted to avoid taking prescription medications. A course of SAM-e partially improved her depression, but it didn't restore her cognitive ability. With the addition of a daily 400-milligram dose of *Rhodiola rosea*, she became more aware and energetic. Dick gradually increased Angela's dosage to 600 milligrams per day, which led to further improvements in her concentration, language skills, mood, and ability to perform at work. For the first time in years, she was able to travel.

Though Angela's recovery is not 100 percent, she successfully copes with stress as it arises. Just as important, she's able to make the most of her life.

ATTENTION DEFICIT DISORDER

Knowing that *Rhodiola rosea* improves attention, concentration, learning, and memory, we've recommended it to patients with attention deficit disorder and dyslexia with good results. This is an exciting area for future research, especially because so many children are being diagnosed with ADD and their parents are concerned about the side effects of prescription medications.

Alice's mother brought her to see Dick when she was 14 years old. She had already been diagnosed with ADD and anxiety—and it was easy to see why. She was so scattered and impulsive that she immediately went to the small bubbling fountain in the office and thrust her hands into the water. During the session, she couldn't sit still. She was up and down, pacing the room.

Not surprisingly, Alice was having difficulty doing her schoolwork and relating to her peers. She had tried various medications, with limited success. And much to her horror, she had gained 25 pounds on Celexa (citalopram), a serotonin reuptake inhibitor.

Dick suggested that Alice try taking 300 milligrams a day of *Rhodiola rosea*. Her schoolwork and organizational skills rapidly improved. She made friends and took up running. A few years later, she went on to college, where she continued to do well.

Alice didn't realize that *Rhodiola rosea* had made such a dramatic difference. Still, her mother gave glowing reports about her daughter's progress, which was evident the day that Alice managed to sit through an entire session without jumping up once.

Like Alice, many young people are successfully treated for ADD in childhood or adolescence. But for some, the right treatment may not come along until much later. This was the case with Jeremy, who sought help at age 27, when he was flunking out of graduate school.

Jeremy had struggled with chronic low-level depression, severe dyslexia, and ADD since childhood. He told Dick that he never felt happy. In fact, he was intensely restless, easily distracted, and filled with self-blame. It wasn't all that surprising that he was failing in graduate school, as well as on the dating front.

Jeremy had tried nearly every medication available for his condition—all with unbearable side effects. A course of SAM-e provided some relief from his depression, but once he added *Rhodiola rosea* to his regimen, he got much better. Within a short time, his mood and energy improved. He was able to focus, complete his work with fewer errors, and—for the first time ever—stop procrastinating.

Wisely, Jeremy left graduate school for a good job. And he became involved in his first long-term relationship.

How to take Rhodiola rosea . . .

FOR A HEALTHY BRAIN

To optimize healthy brain function and minimize deterioration, we make a general recommendation that people over age 40 to take 100 to 400 milligrams of Rhodiola rosea, *plus 1,000 to 3,000 milligrams of omega-3-fatty acids, each day. We also recommend the following:*

vitamin C, vitamin E, and vitamin B-complex, plus separate supplements of vitamin B$_{12}$ and folic acid.

To Improve Memory

Start by taking one 100-milligram capsule of Rhodiola rosea *on an empty stomach ½ hour before breakfast for 1 week. Then add a capsule ½ hour before lunch for 1 week. As long as you are comfortable and experience no agitation, irritability, or sleep disturbance, you can take a second capsule before breakfast for 1 week. Wait several weeks to see the effects. If you feel you need more, add a second capsule before lunch, for a total of four capsules daily.*

For Neurodegenerative Diseases, Brain Injury, and ADD

Start with one 100-milligram capsule of Rhodiola rosea *on an empty stomach ½ hour before breakfast for 3 to 7 days. If you experience no side effects but see no change in your symptoms, then proceed by adding another capsule every 3 to 7 days until you notice improvement or side effects. You may need as much as 600 milligrams a day, though we recommend medical supervision when taking more than 400 milligrams a day.*

In some cases, benefits occur within days; in others, they take 2 or 3 months. So have patience. If by chance you develop side effects, cut back to your previous dosage and increase in smaller increments, so your body has time to adjust. Be sure that your doctor monitors your treatment, especially if you have any other medical condition.

CHAPTER 6

Maximize
PHYSICAL
PERFORMANCE

When Charles Darwin coined the phrase "survival of the fittest" in the mid-19th century, he was referring to those members of each species—including humans—that, for one reason or another, adapt most easily to their environment. This adaptability, he wrote, gives them an edge in surviving long enough to pass on their genetic traits to the next generation.

Darwin took the long view. According to the great scientist—and the biologists who have followed in his footsteps—our genetic makeup doesn't evolve overnight, or even over centuries. It evolves very slowly, over eons and eons.

This puts modern man in a strange new predicament. We're altering our environment so rapidly that our genetic endowment can't possibly keep pace with the social, cultural, and technological changes that are the hallmark of our times. Even though we may be voyaging deep into space, here on earth we still are walking around with many of the same genetic traits as our Stone Age ancestors—including a primitive stress response system. Believe it or not, some features of the human stress response system are reptilian![5]

While our minds keep inventing and adapting, our bodies do not. Their design is ideal for the hunter-gatherer lifestyle, not modern amenities. Just imagine if we still had to sprint to catch our dinner or forage for nuts and berries. None of us would be overweight. Instead, we can kick back in a lounge chair for hours, expending no more effort than is necessary for clicking the remote control or taking an occasional stroll to the refrigerator. The irony is, as we exert less and less physical energy, our energy reserves sink lower and lower. This helps explain why so many of us aren't as healthy as we could be.

The question we humans must ask ourselves is this: What can we do to optimize our chances of successfully adapting to the swiftly changing, fast-paced global village that we now call home? One answer, as we will see, is to increase our physical strength and endurance through exercise and the use of adaptogens—especially *Rhodiola rosea*.

PERSONAL BESTS

Greg, a 45-year-old marathon runner, was looking for a natural supplement to increase his speed and endurance. He had read that *Rhodiola rosea* is effective for enhancing mental and physical stamina, so he decided to try it while training for his next race. Shortly after he started taking the herb, he reported feeling more mentally agile, with fewer dips in his motivation. And he was amazed by the change in his running time. He crossed the finish line in 2 hours, 45 minutes—more than 20 minutes faster than his personal best for any previous marathon.

Rhodiola rosea isn't just for boosting athletic performance. It can prime the body to withstand all manner of challenge, including serious illness. Such was the case with Jack, who sought advice on *Rhodiola rosea* from our good friend Dr. Zakir Ramazanov, an internationally known expert on the herb.

Jack had been mountain climbing and backpacking for 30 years before he could afford to travel and scale the world's highest peaks. At age 51, he conquered Tanzania's 19,300-foot Mount Kilimanjaro. The following year, he began training for a far more rugged trek to the summit of Aconcagua, the 23,000-foot peak in the Andes Mountains.

Jack had heard that *Rhodiola rosea* protects against altitude sickness, so he contacted Zakir, who sent a supply of the root extract. Having been trained as a pharmacist, Jack was able to compound his own capsules, taking 300 milligrams of *Rhodiola rosea* a day. After just 1 week on the herb, he had shaved 5 minutes off his daily 5-mile mountain run. And instead of struggling to catch his breath for several minutes after finishing his workouts, he noticed that his respiration returned to normal within 60 seconds.

Jack was in good form and felt ready to tackle Aconcagua. With a 60-pound pack strapped to his back, he began his ascent from the Argentina side. But as he neared 19,000 feet, he realized that he wasn't going to get to the top. Bitterly disappointed, he turned around and headed back down the mountain.

One month later, a large lump appeared under Jack's arm. Two weeks after that, another lump appeared on his neck. Because he seemed so healthy and showed no other signs of illness, both he and his doctors were shocked to discover that he had stage IV cancer—a rare mantle cell lymphoma with a 1- to 3-year survival rate. When he realized that he had managed to climb to 19,000 feet with advanced cancer, his disappointment over his failed attempt at Aconcagua vanished.

Jack fought cancer with the same intensity and determination with which he had climbed the great peaks of the world. He took megadoses of antioxidants, immune-boosting herbs, Chinese herbal anticancer formulas, and *Rhodiola rosea* as he prepared for experimental cancer chemotherapy, total body irradiation, and a bone marrow transplant. Throughout this grueling course of treatment, he broke every record. He not only produced the largest number of stem cells in the shortest period of time that his doctors had ever seen, he also got discharged the fastest, with a clean bill of health.

Because of his physical stamina and endurance, Jack was able to bounce back from his rigorous treatment regimen and beat an incredibly grim prognosis. He recently surpassed the 3-year mark—the maximum survival rate for his type of cancer—with no sign of the disease. He continues to run and climb and to boost his energy with *Rhodiola rosea* and other supplements.

A BOOST FOR THE MUSCLES

Jack's experience was not a fluke. Beginning in the 1970s, the Soviet Ministry of Health commissioned extensive testing of *Rhodiola rosea* and other adaptogens as energy boosters for Olympic athletes—and got similarly impressive results. In Soviet sports research centers, scientists determined that *Rhodiola rosea* promotes the same kind of muscle-building activity as steroids, only without the negative side effects. (Interestingly, while the International Olympic Committee strictly forbids the use of steroids, Russian athletes routinely take sports formulas containing *Rhodiola rosea* as well as other adaptogens—notably *Eleutherococcus senticosus*, *Panax ginseng*, and *Schizandra chinensis*.)

So how does *Rhodiola rosea* bolster performance? First and foremost, muscles need energy to do their job, and *Rhodiola rosea* stimulates production of the high-energy molecules ATP (adenosine triphosphate) and CP (creatine phosphate) in muscle cells.[1, 6] This increases the amount of energy that's available for greater endurance and faster recovery. It also prevents the cell damage that occurs when oxygen supplies run low.

What's more, research has shown that *Rhodiola rosea* elevates the level of RNA and DNA in muscle cells, leading to increased production of the amino acids and proteins that build and repair muscles through a process called anabolism. In animal studies, the herb has reduced levels of lactic acid and ammonia in tissues, helping to avert muscle fatigue as well as promote synthesis of ATP and CP.[4, 7]

Then, too, *Rhodiola rosea* is antihypoxic. In other words, it improves oxygen utilization in the tissues, which optimizes recovery after exertion. This action is consistent with the long-held view among Russian sports physiologists of exercise as a low-oxygen state, because muscle tissues at work use oxygen at a high rate. By enhancing oxygen's delivery and its uptake by tissues, *Rhodiola rosea* enables athletes to use energy more efficiently, perform with greater strength and endurance, and recover more quickly after exertion.

STRESSED FOR SUCCESS

In the 1990s, under the leadership of Dr. Victor M. Baranov, the Russian Institute of Medical and Biological Problems conducted further research into the impact of herbal adaptogens such as *Rhodiola rosea* on physical performance. Because earlier studies had shown that a well-balanced, flexible autonomic nervous system improved endurance and recovery, Dr. Baranov and his team concentrated on the effects of adaptogens on the autonomic nervous system. (Just to refresh your memory, the sympathetic branch of the autonomic nervous system prepares the body to expend energy by increasing heart rate, respiration, and bloodflow to muscles, while the parasympathetic branch orchestrates recovery and repair during and after exertion.)[3, 5]

Using the ADAPT formula—which contains *Rhodiola rosea*, *Eleutherococus senticosus*, and *Schizandra chinesis*—the researchers conducted numerous double-blind, placebo-controlled trials involving healthy but generally sedentary adult men. In other words, these guys were couch potatoes. The results were impressive. Those who took the adaptogen formula increased their physical work capacity by 28 percent more than those who took a placebo. In fact, in aerobic testing, they could function at the lower levels of trained athletes. This means that even "weekend warriors" and people who do not work out regularly could benefit substantially from *Rhodiola rosea* and other adaptogens.

The ADAPT formula clearly activated the parasympathetic nervous system, improved cardiovascular function, and shortened recovery time in the men who took it. The researchers concluded that the shift in dominance from the sympathetic nervous system to the parasympathetic nervous system induced a state of calm, but with a heightened sense of attention. This is essential for mobilizing energy and maintaining adequate energy reserves while the body is under physical stress. Similar experiments involving cosmonauts during long spaceflights have confirmed these findings.[2]

In effect, adaptogens such as *Rhodiola rosea* benefit physical performance not only by building endurance. They also promote speedy recovery after exertion by helping to optimize the function of the autonomic nervous system.

RHODIOLA ROSEA IN ACTION

As we have seen, *Rhodiola rosea*—either alone or in combination with other adaptogens—can improve physical performance in a laboratory setting. But what about out in the real world, in the heat of competition? The results have held up. Whether running, swimming, speed skating, skiing, weight lifting, wrestling, or performing gymnastics, athletes who took supplements containing *Rhodiola rosea* significantly increased their speed, strength, and endurance.[7, 8]

For one study, researchers recruited 42 healthy male biathletes between ages 20 and 25 and assigned them to one of two groups. Thirty to 60 minutes before a race, one group took an adaptogen formula containing *Rhodiola rosea* and *Eleutherococcus senticosus* extracts, while the other took a placebo. The athletes skied over a 12-mile course, carrying rifles and periodically shooting at targets. Compared with the placebo group, the adaptogen group had better physical endurance and eye-hand coordination, milder arm tremors, and higher shooting scores.

The researchers asked the athletes to perform additional physical tasks at the end of the race, then tested their cardiovascular recovery after 30 minutes. The men who had taken the adaptogen formula measured, on average, between 104 and 106 percent of their prerace heart rates. Among those who had taken the placebo, the figure climbed to an average of 128.7 percent—a difference of 25 percent. This demonstrates that adaptogens not only enhance athletic performance but also shorten recovery time—even in situations of intense competition.

More recent double-blind, placebo-controlled trials focusing on *Rhodiola rosea* have confirmed these promising results. In studies involving students, professionals, and military cadets, those who took the herb showed significant improvements over those who took placebos, as reflected in several key measures, including cardiovascular function, neuromotor skills, blood pressure, physical fitness, and general well-being.[9, 10, 11] This certainly was the case with George, a 52-year-old patient of Dick's.

Although George was a lifelong athlete who enjoyed rowing,

boxing, and weight training, he felt so depleted after his mornings at the gym that he seriously considered giving up his workouts altogether. The very thought depressed him, but he was convinced that he didn't have a choice—until a course of *Rhodiola rosea*, 400 milligrams a day, restored his strength and energy. In fact, George reported that beyond feeling more pumped up for his workouts, he was more clearheaded and energetic throughout the day. His relationships at home and at work improved as well.

Whether your goal is to get more from your exercise routine or to compete at the highest levels of your chosen sport, you can find safe, high-quality supplements to maximize your physical performance. You can mix and match individual adaptogens to meet your needs, or you can choose from among the many commercially available sports formulas. Some of the best products contain *Rhodiola rosea*. We'll discuss our recommendations at the end of this chapter.

HERBAL HELP FOR GENETIC DISORDERS

From time to time, we see patients with rare genetic disorders that cause abnormally weak muscles (muscular dystrophy) or unusually lax tendons (Ehlers-Danlos syndrome). For these people, weakness, fatigue, and lack of energy are constant companions. They come to us not for relief from their physical symptoms but for treatment of depression and anxiety.

Those with medical problems that affect their physical function often exhibit unique body chemistry and so may experience adverse reactions to standard medications such as antidepressants and anti-anxiety drugs. Since adaptogens like *Rhodiola rosea* offer a broad range of benefits with few side effects, we feel that they're worth trying. By presenting two such case studies from our practices, we hope to generate interest in alternative treatments for these progressive, debilitating disorders, for which there currently is no cure.

Paul is a 29-year-old computer programmer who loves nature and bird watching. He has muscular dystrophy, a genetic disorder that affects his muscles' energy metabolism. Ever since childhood, he has been adapting to the physical and psychological stresses of a progressive muscle weakness that affects his mobility, endurance, and recovery from exertion. In people with muscular dystrophy, numbness, stiffness, twitching, and muscle spasms also are common.

Over the years, Paul's devout faith, strong friendships, and devilish sense of humor had gotten him through many tough times. But he was feeling fearful and depressed when he sought help from Pat. Although he worried about taking medication—he had experienced unusual side effects from so many others—he agreed to try SAM-e. While it relieved his joint pain and muscle stiffness as well as his depression, it also increased his irritability and mood swings. Consequently, he could take only 400 milligrams of SAM-e a day, which is a low dose.

With the addition of 100 milligrams of *Rhodiola rosea* twice a day, Paul got much better. After 1 month on the herb, he couldn't stop smiling. *Rhodiola rosea* had balanced his mood, so he was on an even keel. His energy increased, and the annoying nighttime muscle spasms stopped. Paul found that he could work longer hours without getting tired and could recover faster than before. As a bonus, his libido—and his interest in women—returned.

Unfortunately, like the rest of Paul's muscles, his heart muscle was weakening as a result of his illness. To complicate matters, the medications prescribed for his heart condition left him so exhausted that he could barely function, even on half the recommended doses. *Rhodiola rosea* once again came to the rescue, helping to relieve his medication-induced fatigue.

Perhaps the most surprising change was that after more than 10 years, Paul began dreaming again. He knew that dreams occur during a phase of deep sleep called REM (rapid eye movement), when the body restores energy reserves. Paul surmised that during all his dreamless years, he had been missing out on this natural recovery process. He was thrilled to recover his ability to dream and to wake up truly refreshed, with enough energy to get out of bed and make the most of the day ahead.

Naomi had Ehlers-Danlos syndrome, a genetic disorder that affects the connective tissues. As a result, her tendons were so loose that she repeatedly dislocated most of the joints in her body, including her fingers, arms, shoulders, hips, ankles, and knees. Sometimes she felt like the scarecrow in the *Wizard of Oz*. But since she was not made of straw, she risked serious injury every time she fell down.

Naomi also suffered from Sjögren's syndrome—an autoimmune disease that causes joint inflammation, pain, and dry eyes—as well as fibromyalgia, insomnia, and severe chronic fatigue. Still, she possessed a fighting spirit and a world-class sense of humor. These attributes certainly helped as she earned her master's degree and pursued a successful 15-year career in social services. Then her medical problems became just too debilitating.

When Naomi first limped into Pat's office, she was fearful, depressed, and exhausted. She constantly worried about the future, which sent her stress level off the charts. And she was dogged by fatigue and nausea—side effects of all the medications that she was taking.

The first phase of treatment—which included psychotherapy, neurotherapy (an advanced form of biofeedback), photon stimulation (a new technique for relieving pain and inflammation), and medication—reduced Naomi's anxiety and physical pain. Remeron (mirtazapine)—an antidepressant with stomach-calming action—helped to relieve her nausea. Next, she wanted to try *Rhodiola rosea* for her fatigue. As her dosage of the herb increased, so did her level of energy. With 600 milligrams daily, she felt an energy surge that pushed her to walk twice as far as she could before. Instead of looking to the future with dread, she began to feel more optimistic.

Today Naomi is much more relaxed than before. And she's better able to manage her multiple medical problems without feeling panicked or overwhelmed.

How to take Rhodiola rosea . . .

TO IMPROVE PHYSICAL STRENGTH, ENDURANCE, AND PERFORMANCE

As we mentioned earlier, many good adaptogen-based sports formulas are available commercially. Which one you choose depends on how healthy you are and how intensely you work out. Here we offer four examples of quality brands. The first two, Synergy and Prime One, are intended for use as daily supplements to a healthful diet. The second two, Optygen and Second Wind, are designed for competitive athletes. (For more advice on creating an energizing supplement regimen, see chapter 15.)

- *Synergy combines* Rhodiola rosea, Eleutherococcus senticosus, Schizandra chinesis, Rhaponticum carthamoides, *and* Aralia mandshurica.

- *Prime One contains the same five herbs, plus* Glycyrrhiza uralensis *(Ural licorice root),* Rosa majalis *(cinnamon rose), and MA complex (adaptogens plus molasses and food additives).*

- *Optygen contains 300 milligrams of* Rhodiola rosea, *1,000 milligrams of* Cordyceps sinensis CS-4, *200 milligrams of chromium (which helps to regulate glucose metabolism and insulin), and a proprietary mixture of calcium, pyruvate, sodium phosphate, potassium phosphate, ribose, and adenosine.*

- *Second Wind, an alternative to Optygen, is made from* Panax ginseng, Eleutherococus senticosus, *cordyceps, enoki and reishi mushroom extracts, and citrus peel extract. It does not contain* Rhodiola rosea, *but you can take the herb as a separate supplement, if you wish.*

For someone whose regular physical activities include moderate exercise such as brisk walking or biking for 20 to 30 minutes a day, we recommend a daily regimen of two to four 100-milligram capsules of Rhodiola rosea. *We also suggest a good multivitamin such as Geriforte or Bio-Strath for extra B vitamins, minerals, and antioxidants.*

People who engage in intense aerobic workouts or weight training, or who participate in competitive sports, need stronger formulas. So do those whose jobs require sudden intense physical exertion, such as police, firemen, military personnel, ski patrol members, mechanics, and construction workers. For them, we recommend a combination of three supplements: Geriforte; Synergy or Prime 1; and Optygen or Second Wind.

Many of us lose muscle mass as we get older, mostly because of inactivity and hormonal changes. Prolonged inactivity after surgery or illness can have the same effect. For those over age 45, we suggest the following regimen: Geriforte; Synergy; and Rhodiola rosea, *starting with one 100-milligram capsule and increasing slowly, as tolerated, to a maximum of four capsules a day.*

CHAPTER 7

Extreme
STRESS:
THE FINAL FRONTIER

Space is the ultimate extreme environment for testing human performance under stress. Astronauts must endure hypergravity during launch and weightlessness during flight—not to mention confinement in cramped quarters, lack of privacy, and a heavy physical and mental workload. Long hours of tedium may be interrupted by dangerous crises, such as equipment failures.

Extravehicular activities—including transfers into and out of the ship, as well as space walks—are the most stressful parts of missions. The combination of intense physical effort, emotional strain, and disorientation can raise the pulse to as high as 154 beats a minute.[8]

On the interpersonal front, interactions between team members can be charged, even when things are proceeding according to plan. Not surprisingly, the sheer magnitude of social and psychological stresses that astronauts must deal with from the moment of liftoff can result in depression, insomnia, irritability, and poor judgment. Failure to adapt emotionally and physically can endanger the life of everyone on board.[6, 7, 11]

The hazards of mental stress during space missions became evident soon after man first struck out to explore the heavens. NASA uses the word *off-nominal* to euphemistically describe maladaptive behaviors among its astronauts. These breaches may include anything from violation of safety procedures and insubordination to poor judgment and insensitivity to fellow crew members.

Although the stresses of space exploration are more extreme than the stresses of our earthbound existence, they have many similarities and therefore can provide valuable insights into the physical and psychological implications of stress. Many of the physical changes that occur in space, such as loss of bone density and muscle mass as well as declines in the neuroendocrine system, are similar to those that occur with aging. If adaptogen formulas containing *Rhodiola rosea* are powerful enough to help astronauts overcome stress, imagine what they could do for you.

The Odd Couple

In 1982, two Soviet cosmonauts, Anatoly Berezovoi (Tolia) and Valentin Lebedvev (Valia), spent 7 months together on the *Salyut 7* space station. Not surprisingly, they started getting on each other's nerves. Valia—annoyed at having to catch cameras as they floated around due to lack of gravity—decided that the equipment was Tolia's responsibility, irritating his crewmate. After arguing, the two men agreed to create a wall inside the space station using a piece of scrap metal as a partition.

As they proceeded to cut, metal shavings flew in every direction, one of them lodging in Valia's eye. This was a wake-up call for both men. They realized that if they couldn't remove the shard, they would be forced to abort their mission and return to Earth.

Luckily, Tolia was able to clear Valia's eye, and the two men completed their mission. But this off-nominal incident clearly shows how extreme stress can lead two highly trained individuals to take unnecessary risks.[4]

THE ILL-FATED SPEKTR

During the Cold War, the Soviet Ministry of Defense developed the *Spektr* space module as part of a top-secret military program code named Oktant. *Spektr*'s intended mission was to dock at the *Mir* orbiting space station with its load of surveillance equipment and launchers for antimissile defense. But as the arms race wound down, the ship never left the ground.

After the Cold War, *Spektr* got a new lease on life with an overhaul for use in the joint U.S.–Russian space program. The space module traveled to *Mir* with experimental equipment and solar panels to supplement the aging solar arrays on the space station, which at the time had been orbiting Earth for more than 10 years. *Spektr* docked in one of *Mir*'s six ports. A Russian shuttle craft called *Soyuz*, which had transported crew members to the space station, sat in another.

On September 25, 1997, U.S. astronaut Mike Foale was aboard *Mir* with two Russian cosmonauts, Commander Vasily Tsibliev and Alexander Lazutkin, when a potentially catastrophic collision occurred. Tsibliev had been guiding an unmanned supply ship, the *Progress*, to one of *Mir*'s ports. The *Progress* struck *Spektr*, causing it to leak air and depressurize the entire space station.

The crew saved itself by sealing the hatch between *Spektr* and *Mir*, then repressurizing the space station. Unfortunately, they failed to notice that they were rapidly losing energy in their reserve batteries. The collision had spun *Mir* off-course; its solar panels were facing away from the sun and no longer collecting energy.

Eventually, the space station lost all power. The crew was left with no lights and no life-support systems. Foale described the harrowing events: "We had used up all the reserve energy. . . . There was nothing on. This lasted . . . 30 hours. . . . It was the hardest time I ever had on the station. . . . We got so tired. . . . We were spinning."[5]

In a brief radio transmission, mission control advised the crew to use the engines of the *Soyuz* shuttle to correct their spin and reposition *Mir*. Then all contact was lost. No one on *Mir* knew how to alter the spin of the space station. To make matters worse, the crew didn't know how much they should spin, what axis they should spin on, or where *Mir* was in relation to the sun, which they couldn't see.

As the level of carbon dioxide built up inside the module, Foale, a physicist, made his best calculations. He felt a terrible responsibility for the crew; he worried that if they used too much of *Soyuz*'s fuel, they wouldn't have any way of getting back to Earth. They would endlessly spin in space.

During those dark hours, the three men devised a plan. Tsibliev transferred to *Soyuz*, and Foale instructed him to fire a thruster. Tsibliev worried about using up precious fuel, but Foale persuaded him to fire for 3 seconds—just long enough to change *Mir*'s direction. The men watched through a window as the stars passed by, and then the sun appeared. Once pointed toward the sun, the solar arrays began collecting the necessary energy to recharge the space station's batteries.

THE SEARCH FOR SPOCK

Anecdotes like these from the annals of space exploration convey the intensity of the physical, mental, and emotional stress that await us on the journey to the final frontier. The ideal astronaut would be mentally alert at all times and completely unaffected by stress or emotion—in other words, Mr. Spock. But alas, we humans are not as unflappable as the Vulcans of *Star Trek*.

Early in the development of their space program, the Soviets realized that the success of their missions depended on the ability of their cosmonauts to overcome extreme stress and function as team players. With this in mind, the Institute of Medical and Biological Problems (IMBP)—under the direction of Dr. Victor M. Baranov—extensively tested the adaptogen formula ADAPT, a blend of *Rhodiola rosea*, *Schizandra chinesis*, and *Eleutherococcus senticosus*. The hope was that the formula (also known as MPPA, which stands for mono- and polyphenolic acids) would improve alertness and resistance to stress. As Dr. Baranov wrote, "The search for ways to maintain high mental and professional working capacity of cosmonauts at all stages of a long-term flight is the most important task of space psychology."[1]

In order to evaluate the potential of MPPA, Dr. Baranov and his team chose male technology students and engineers—a highly motivated, competitive group. Half of the study participants took the formula, while the rest took a placebo. About 12 hours into a 24-hour period of continuous repetitive work requiring a high level of attention, the men in the placebo group had developed a somewhat negative attitude toward their assigned task. At the end of 24 hours, they showed even greater negativity, as well as diminished motivation.

In contrast, the men in the MPPA group were better able to hold their focus through 12 hours of work. After 24 hours, their outlook remained positive. What's more, they managed to maintain a high level of productivity throughout the tests and even to find satisfaction in completing the tedious work.[1] The adaptogen formula clearly improved mental function as well, as demonstrated by enhanced alertness, abstract thinking, reaction time, and short-term memory. The men taking MPPA made half as many mistakes as those taking the placebo.[1]

As Dr. Baranov wrote, "The study of psychoemotional states shows that the effect of the adaptogen was most evident in emotionally labile subjects (those who are prone to becoming upset, overreacting, or experiencing emotional extremes) with insufficient stress resistance. Adaptogen treatment changes positively their perception of the experiment conditions, their attitude toward work, and their self-evaluation. . . . Herbal adaptogens are a reliable means for optimizing the psychophysiological state and working capacity of operators in extreme conditions, especially during long work at night."[1]

ADAPTOGENS IMPROVE STRESS RESPONSE

One way in which the adaptogen formula made a difference for the study participants who took it was by improving the function of the autonomic nervous system, both at rest and under physical stress. The outcome of Dr. Baranov's research supports the idea that adaptogens help to balance the sympathetic, or reactive, branch of the autonomic nervous system with the calming and recharging parasympathetic branch, especially during the recovery period after mental and physical exertion. Adaptogens also act on the part of the stress response system called the hypothalamic-pituitary-adrenal axis. Dr. Baranov concluded his report by recommending the MPPA formula for use in space flights to improve stress resistance.[2]

Studies of long-term confinement—the norm during space missions—show that men experience significant increases in epinephrine and norepinephrine secretion, especially during stressful changes in group dynamics.[9] The rise in these stress hormones indicates increased activity of the sympathetic nervous system and the part of the HPA axis that releases epinephrine from the adrenal medulla. On a psychological level, a person might feel more tense, anxious, and irritable, with difficulty relaxing. The physical effects could include a more rapid heart rate and increased strain on the heart.

The potential for stressful interpersonal conflicts and misunderstandings is a growing safety concern for space programs as crews become larger and more multinational. How well individual crew members adapt to their situations, both physically and psychologically, directly influences how well they execute their missions.

WILL WE EVER KNOW?

So, did the Russian space program accept Dr. Baranov's recommendation? Did they give the adaptogen formula to cosmonauts in missions conducted during and after 1994, the year that Dr. Baranov submitted his report? We suspected that they did, given their concerns about the dangers inherent in space travel and the strong evidence of adaptogens' benefits under such extreme conditions. But until recently, we couldn't be certain. The Russians maintained a high level of secrecy, even during their joint collaborations with NASA on space station *Mir*.

For this reason, finding evidence that the Russian cosmonauts used MPPA in their space missions wasn't easy. But after months of seeking information from every imaginable source, Pat got the break she was hoping for when the Swedish Herbal Institute sent a pile of research reports. Among the documents were abstracts of lectures from a seminar on adaptogens in Gothenburg, Sweden, on November 4 and 5, 1996—including a two-paragraph abstract of Dr. Valery Polyakov's presentation, "The Use of a New Phytoadaptogen under Conditions of Space Flight."[12]

Dr. Polyakov was the famous physician-cosmonaut who spent 8 months aboard *Mir* in 1989 and returned in 1994 to set the world record for spaceflight—437 days in orbit. Once, when a fire broke out on the space station, he smothered it with space suits and then prayed with his icon of the Virgin Mary and Child. He later became deputy director of the IMBP, taking part in more missions and testing new methods for providing medical assistance in space.

Dr. Polyakov stayed on *Mir* from January 1994 until March 1995, conducting more research on the effects of spaceflight on the human body. We believe that one of his projects involved testing the ADAPT formula. The first clue appeared in one of Dr. Baranov's 1994 reports, in which he compared his findings with those of tests performed on cosmonauts in space. Where else besides *Mir* could these tests have taken place?

The final proof appeared in the abstract of Dr. Polyakov's lecture at the Gothenburg seminar. There he presented the results of extensive, complex studies of ADAPT, which he concluded by recommending the formula for use during spaceflight under a doctor's supervision. In his report, Dr. Polyakov confirmed that the adaptogen formula had been tested on cosmonauts during preflight training and on board *Mir*, with positive effects on their general well-being. Specifically, it reduced fatigue—especially during the evening hours—and prolonged the cosmonauts' working time. And as Dr. Polyakov noted, "It also optimized their ability to endure the changes in (the) gas atmosphere of the spaceship."[12] Undoubtedly, he was the one who had conducted the studies of ADAPT during his 1994 visit to *Mir*.

Dr. Polyakov spent 437 days on *Mir* to prove that man could survive a trip to Mars. In fact, Dr. Polyakov once asked John Glenn if he would consider traveling to the Red Planet, to which the veteran astronaut replied, "With you, Valery, anytime."[10]

LESSONS FROM SPACE

The disruption of appetite, sleep, and normal physiological processes during extreme stress contributes to anxiety and depression, especially in space. These problems become more severe as missions become longer. Studies of animals and humans in simulated or actual space-flight have documented changes in neuroendocrine, cardiovascular, and immune response. Interestingly, as mentioned earlier, some of these changes are similar to the processes that occur as we grow older—underscoring the potential of adaptogens to help counteract the effects of aging.

The extreme stress of spaceflight also may inhibit reproduction. In one study, a group of female Japanese quails sent to *Mir* stopped laying eggs. Eight days after returning to Earth, they started laying again. Researchers determined that the quails reacted to the physical stress of the launch, as well as to weightlessness in space. In a separate study, a joint Russian-Swedish project called Interstam AM, Japanese quails were subjected to simulated spaceflight. The birds who were kept on their normal diets stopped laying eggs, while those that were fed the ADAPT formula continued laying. The researchers concluded that the adaptogens reduced the quails' excitability and dampened their negative response to stress.[3]

This particular adaptogen benefit may be of use in the future. On long intergalactic missions, we humans may need to reproduce in space, even if we manage to attain warp speed!

EARTHLY IMPLICATIONS

Any living creatures sent into space—humans as well as quails—encounter the most physically and psychologically challenging circumstances imaginable. Yet space travel is only one example of a work environment where human error in the face of stress can take a tremendous toll. Just think back to 1979, when employee missteps during an overnight shift at the Three Mile Island nuclear power plant contributed to the most serious nuclear accident in U.S. history—one that came perilously close to a full-blown nuclear disaster.

Clearly, life on Earth has its extreme stresses, too. The potential uses of *Rhodiola rosea*, either alone or in a formula with other adaptogens, are as plentiful as high-stress jobs. Air traffic controllers, pilots, military defense monitors, submarine crews, heavy equipment operators, policemen, firemen, doctors and nurses, emergency medical technicians, even everyday highway commuters must endure long hours of tiring work punctuated by unpredictable crises that require split-second decisions. Alertness, attention, and a well-tuned stress response system can mean the difference between life and death.

Regardless of the stresses that confront you on the job or at home, the benefits of adaptogens like *Rhodiola rosea*—improved stress tolerance, fewer errors, a more positive attitude—will enhance your mental and physical performance as well as your quality of life. And you don't need to sign up for the next space mission to discover the therapeutic power of this remarkable herb!

CHAPTER 8

SAFEGUARD
YOUR HEART

Think for a moment of the eloquent expressions that we use to describe our hearts. They may be full of love or heavy with sorrow. They may bleed. Sometimes they feel as though they're pounding against our ribs or they've skipped a beat. We say that our hearts rise into our throats or drop to our feet, as though they've broken free of their moorings.

When we are sincere, our words are heartfelt. If we give our love to someone who's untrue, our hearts ache or break. Of course, when we find a new sweetheart, we don't mind if our old flames eat their hearts out.

Metaphors like these capture a simple truth: The heart is exquisitely sensitive to emotion and stress. Science explains that both branches of the autonomic nervous system act directly on the heart, which is essential during the fight-or-flight response. Whether we're physically threatened, emotionally agitated, or sexually aroused, the body's stress response system kicks into gear and releases cortisol, epinephrine (adrenaline), and norepinephrine. These "stress hormones" help speed up the heart and increase the amount of blood and oxygen being pumped through the coronary arteries. The muscle cells of the heart must produce enough energy to beat faster and stronger, supporting whatever action may be necessary—fending off an attack, running for safety, or making love.

Every aspect of heart function, from the condition of coronary arteries and heart muscle cells to the transmission of electrical impulses that regulate heartbeat, is under the influence of the stress response system. In cases of severe or chronic stress, the sustained release of stress hormones—which normally would help save our lives in an emergency—instead turns against our bodies and damages our organs, including our hearts. Given that heart disease ranks as the number one killer of American men and women, the wear and tear on a heart under stress is cause for serious concern.

WHAT THE HEART NEEDS MOST

Rhodiola rosea can enhance heart function. First and foremost, it works by helping to restore balance in the autonomic nervous system—specifically, by curtailing the reactivity of the sympathetic branch while strengthening the calming and recharging action of the parasympathetic branch.

In chapter 2, we talked at length about the role of the vagus nerve in the calming action of the parasympathetic nervous system. To summarize, the more active the vagus nerve, the slower the heart rate, which reduces the likelihood of an irregular heartbeat. This is reflected in improved heart rate variability (HRV) and energy efficiency, as well as increased energy reserves.[2]

HRV uses frequencies emitted by a beating heart to analyze the normal variations in heart rate that occur with breathing, changes in oxygen and body temperature, and other factors. The high frequencies can help measure vagus nerve activity. Recent research has shown a strong link between HRV, stress, and the outcome of myocardial infarction, or heart attack. Specifically, an increase in the high frequencies of HRV—indicating vagus nerve action on the heart—appears to not only lower the risk of cardiovascular disease but also improve the odds of surviving a heart attack[5] and the speed of recovery.[8] By supporting the parasympathetic nervous system, and thus the vagus nerve, *Rhodiola rosea* promotes heart health.

Restoring balance to the autonomic nervous system has other important benefits for the heart. For example, a slower heart rate—brought on by the calming action of the parasympathetic nervous system—means less demand for oxygen and a lower risk of damage from hypoxia, or reduced oxygen flow. This is critical when you consider that depriving the heart muscle of its blood supply, and thus oxygen, can result in angina or a heart attack. The word *angina* refers to the pain that occurs when the heart muscle cells don't get enough oxygen. If a shortage of oxygen lasts too long, it can damage or destroy the heart muscle cells, leading to a heart attack.

The loss of blood supply, a condition called ischemia, often occurs when the atherosclerotic plaques commonly associated with high cholesterol narrow the coronary arteries. Anything that helps protect the heart muscle from the temporary loss of blood supply—or that supports the healing of heart tissue compromised by the lack of oxygen—increases the chances of preventing a heart attack as well as surviving or recovering from one. *Rhodiola rosea* appears to be up to the task. When researchers gave the herb to laboratory animals for 8 days prior to the onset of experimental ischemia, the heart muscle resisted damage and recovered strength and tone far better than in animals not given the herb.[1]

If atherosclerosis disrupts bloodflow to certain areas of the brain, it can trigger what's known as a transient ischemic attack (TIA). Common symptoms of a TIA include temporary loss of speech, loss of consciousness, and paralysis on one side of the face or body. The loss of blood supply during a TIA can damage nerve cells. And once bloodflow is restored—a process called reperfusion—swelling and biochemical reactions can cause further harm. In a recent animal study, *Rhodiola rosea* prevented brain injury, swelling, and oxidative damage in animals with experimental cerebral ischemia.[4]

Other animal studies involving *Rhodiola rosea* hint at even greater protective effects for the heart.[3] For example, the herb prevents damage to heart muscle cells by increasing cellular production of energy and the synthesis of proteins.[1, 6, 7, 9] It also guards against the excessive release of epinephrine and norepinephrine by the sympathetic nervous system, which can cause rapid heart rate or irregular heartbeat.

More clinical trials are necessary to assess just how these cardioprotective effects might play out in humans. The outcome of such research should reinforce *Rhodiola rosea*'s growing reputation as a guardian of heart health.

THE HERB AT WORK

Matt, an advertising executive, suffered from constant anxiety—a situation made worse by heart disease and fluctuating blood pressure. By the time he turned 52, Matt had undergone three angioplasties to reopen his clogged coronary arteries. He also had experienced a minor transient ischemic attack, with temporary loss of bloodflow to a small area of his brain.

Although he recovered completely from the TIA, Matt feared further episodes—or worse. Between his poor health and his anxiety, he felt sluggish, apathetic, and too fearful and distracted to meet his deadlines at work.

Matt was 63 when he consulted Dick, who prescribed a small dose of *Rhodiola rosea*—just 50 milligrams a day. That was enough to improve his energy, mood, and capacity for exercise while diminishing his anxiety. Now he spends less time worrying and more time enjoying life.

People with high blood pressure also can benefit from *Rhodiola rosea*. Another of Dick's patients, a 47-year-old building contractor named Ken, is the perfect case in point.

When Ken first sought Dick's help, his blood pressure—taken during an annual physical exam for his life insurance coverage—measured 188/112. (For comparison, a normal reading is 120/80.) He had switched to a low-salt diet on the advice of his doctor, but his numbers kept climbing. He also had tried blood pressure medication, but he suffered unbearable side effects.

Ken worried that if his blood pressure didn't come down, his insurance rates would go up—something he could ill afford with twins about to enter college. Making matters worse, he had begun to experience full-blown panic attacks, characterized by extreme apprehension, severe headache, heavy perspiration, and rapid heartbeat. These episodes would start abruptly and last 10 to 15 minutes.

Dick prescribed *Rhodiola rosea*—100 milligrams three times a day. Almost immediately, Ken's apprehension began to diminish. After 1 month on the herb, he reported no further anxiety attacks; after 6 months, he was symptom-free. Ken was thrilled when, at his most recent annual physical, he learned that his blood pressure had dropped to 118/78.

How to take Rhodiola rosea . . .

FOR HIGH BLOOD PRESSURE

If you're taking medication for high blood pressure, don't throw away your pills. First talk to your doctor about trying Rhodiola rosea *in conjunction with your regular medication. Start with 100 milligrams ½ hour before breakfast for the first week. If all goes well, add another 100 milligrams ½ hour before lunch for the second week. If you still encounter no problems, increase your dosage to 200 milligrams before breakfast and continue with the 100 milligrams before lunch.*

Stay at this dosage for at least a month before rechecking your blood pressure. If necessary, you may add another 100 milligrams before lunch, for a total of 400 milligrams a day. If you experience a significant decline in blood pressure with this regimen, then you and your doctor can discuss gradually reducing your antihypertensive medication. Rhodiola rosea *does not work in all cases, but it is particularly helpful when stress, anxiety, and depression contribute to high blood pressure.*

FOR HEART TROUBLE

If you have a heart condition, talk to your doctor about taking Rhodiola rosea. *She may want to learn more about the herb to determine the best way to use it in your situation. Direct her to the references for this chapter (see page 239); the articles there should provide the information she needs.*

The safest bet is to start with a small dose and wait a week before increasing it. If you experience any agitation or other symptoms, cut back to the previous dose, or even to a fraction of a capsule. You may need more time at the lower dose. Some people do best when they step up their dosages gradually.

CHAPTER 9

Lift a

BLUE

OR ANXIOUS MOOD

For 20 years, Maria, a stay-at-home mom, fought a losing battle with depression. Even the simplest tasks became a struggle as she sank deeper and deeper into the quicksand of her illness. She not only cut herself off from the network of mothers who had once been her support system, but she also began napping for hours during the day, missing out on precious time with her family.

Eventually, at the urging of her husband, Maria sought help from a psychiatrist, who prescribed a series of antidepressants. None of them worked. Eventually, the marriage failed, and Maria's husband filed for divorce. Though his decision sent her into a tailspin at first, over time, she grew even more determined to get well for the sake of her children.

On the advice of a friend, Maria tried *Rhodiola rosea*. Within a few weeks, her depression began to lift. Not long after, she tossed her medication in the trash, continuing to take 100 milligrams of the herb three times a day.

Maria forged healthy relationships with her children and deepened her ties to family and friends. Today she reports feeling happier and more actively engaged in her life. She even has ventured into dating once again.

THE HERBAL MOOD BOOSTER

Only a small number of clinical trials have evaluated *Rhodiola rosea* as a treatment for depression, anxiety, and post-traumatic stress disorder. But we have seen so many patients like Maria respond remarkably well to the herb that we consider it an important addition to the pharmacopoeia for mood and anxiety disorders.

Until we began working with *Rhodiola rosea*, we were troubled by the fact that many patients taking prescription antidepressants never seemed to get as well as we believed they could.[7] Even if they did improve, all too often they couldn't tolerate the side effects of the drugs. We continue to use medications in our practice because they can help to manage the symptoms of mood disorders so people can reclaim their lives. What bothered us is that while symptoms may subside, they seldom go away completely. Our patients described themselves as not exactly depressed or anxious, but not really happy either.

This is where *Rhodiola rosea* can make a dramatic difference. The herb seems to add spice to life—feelings of joy, pleasure, and excitement. Many formerly depressed or anxious patients have told us how *Rhodiola rosea* has enabled them to be happy again, to connect with other people, to feel grounded. The side effects, if any, tend to be extremely mild; in our experience, very few people are unable to tolerate them.

Although more research is necessary, the positive effects of *Rhodiola rosea* on depression and other mood disorders are not surprising. To begin with, by helping to calm an overactive stress response system and replenish depleted energy reserves, the herb enhances our ability to tolerate stress—the primary cause of depression and anxiety. And just like conventional antidepressants, *Rhodiola rosea* boosts the levels of neurotransmitters that play a critical role in regulating mood, energy, and the ability to enjoy life—only without the negative side effects.

In recent studies, scientists have determined that besides acting on neurotransmitters, antidepressants affect the hypothalamic-pituitary-adrenal axis—an essential component of the stress response system. *Rhodiola rosea* does the exact same thing. So it stands to scientific reason that the herb and its pharmaceutical counterparts would share many of the same benefits.

WHAT THE RESEARCH SHOWS

In the 1970s and 1980s, a few studies of *Rhodiola rosea* as a treatment for depression were published in the Soviet Union. Although these studies don't meet all the modern criteria for scientifically rigorous research, they do provide valuable clinical observations about the herb's therapeutic value.

For example, in a group of 128 adult patients with depression and neurasthenia (a general term for patients with fatigue, weakness, and the inability to recover by resting), treatment with 150 milligrams of *Rhodiola rosea* three times a day significantly reduced or eliminated symptoms in 64 percent of the study participants.[8] And among a group of patients hospitalized for depression, the addition of *Rhodiola rosea* to a treatment regimen of tricyclic antidepressants reduced the length of hospital stays—as well as improved the patients' mood, thought processes, and motor activity. Even better, the herb not only appeared to reduce the troublesome side effects of antidepressants, but it also proved effective in treating less severe forms of depression without other medications.[5]

So why have so few studies examined *Rhodiola rosea* as a treatment for depression and other mood disorders? We don't know for sure, but we suspect that in the former Soviet Union—where the government controlled all the scientific research—the priority was to improve physical and mental performance, especially in competitive fields such as science, space exploration, and military development. Mental illness simply wasn't on the radar screen. So despite the very promising results of early studies, scientists didn't pursue this aspect of research until after the collapse of the communist regime.

Since the 1990s, renewed interest in reducing psychological stress finally has pushed *Rhodiola rosea* to the forefront of scientific exploration. In all of the studies to date, the herb has significantly lessened mental stress and anxiety while enhancing mood and intellectual performance. For example, in one study of Indian students—90 percent of whom experienced difficult adjustment periods and overwhelming fatigue during their first year in Russia—those taking 50 milligrams of *Rhodiola rosea* twice a day reported significantly improved mood and motivation compared with those taking a placebo.[10]

DEPRESSION: AN UNCHECKED EPIDEMIC

Depression, which doctors sometimes describe as the common cold of psychiatric disorders, affects about 121 million people worldwide. It is the leading cause of disability when measured in terms of lost workdays and income.

In the United States alone, major depression afflicts more than 17 million people each year. In fact, adults living in America have a 30 percent chance of experiencing major depression at some point in their lifetimes. The risk rises to a staggering 50 percent for milder forms of depression. And the numbers are skyrocketing: The World Health Organization estimates that by 2020, depression will be second only to heart disease in its impact on global health.[12]

Although the symptoms—low energy, low or flat mood, disturbed sleep or eating habits, poor concentration, guilt or low self-esteem, loss of interest and pleasure in life—are well known, depression remains one of the most underdiagnosed disorders on earth. Tragically, fewer than 25 percent of people with the disorder—and in some countries fewer than 10 percent—have access to adequate treatment. Lack of financial resources and trained providers, coupled with the social stigma still attached to depression, persist as barriers to care.

Who's most likely to develop depression? Age and gender certainly play deciding roles. The disorder is two to three times more common in the elderly than in the young, and twice as likely to affect women as men.

A recent Swedish study of women with and without coronary artery disease identified marital stress as a significant contributing factor to the incidence of depression in the female population.[1] It isn't that men aren't devastated by failed relationships—they frequently are—but women are more likely to become seriously depressed for longer periods of time. The divorce rate, which currently stands at 50 percent in industrialized nations, is one obvious reason for the prevalence of depression among women. So is the stress brought on by the unprecedented pressures and responsibilities of trying to juggle family and career.

Although depression is more common in women and the elderly, its impact is more lethal in young men. In the United States, suicide is the third leading cause of death among men between ages 15 and 25. Those in minority groups, particularly young Latinos, seem especially likely to suffer from depression or contemplate suicide.[6] Long separations from family members left behind in native countries are thought to play a significant role.

Incidentally, while we Americans tend to view depression as a by-product of living in a modern industrialized society, indigenous peoples worldwide are suffering, too. Many factors—war, famine, geographic dislocation, and the destruction of tribal cultures—are having disastrous effects on the mental health of native populations.

THE ANTIDEPRESSANT QUANDARY

Over the past 40 years, Western psychiatry has subdivided depression into many categories, ranging from mild adjustment disorder with de-

---

What Is Major Depression?

Major depression is a psychiatric diagnosis based on one or more major depressive episodes. To qualify as a major depressive episode, it must meet three criteria:

1. At least five of the following symptoms must be present during the same 2-week period, with either depressed mood or loss of interest as one of the five. In addition, each symptom must represent a change from previous function.

- Depressed mood most of the day (for example, feeling sad or empty)
- Markedly diminished interest or pleasure in nearly all activities most of the day
- Fatigue or loss of energy nearly every day
- Significant unintended weight loss or gain (more than 5 percent of body weight per month)
- Insomnia or hypersomnia (excessive sleeping) nearly every day
- Observable psychomotor agitation (restless, nervousness, inability to sit still) or retardation (mental and physical slowness)

---

pressed mood to severe major depression with psychotic features. Regardless of the subtleties of diagnosis, three of the factors that contribute to depression are an overactive stress response system, depleted energy reserves, and inadequate recharging by the parasympathetic branch of the autonomic nervous system.

Doctors treat most cases of depression—whether triggered by neurochemical, genetic, or situational causes—with some form of antidepressant medication. These drugs—which include Effexor (venlafaxine), Wellbutrin (bupropion), and selective serotonin reuptake inhibitors such as Prozac (fluoxetine) and Zoloft (sertraline), among others—correct neurochemical imbalances and improve nerve cell function. The good news is that these medications, in combination with psychotherapy, can help the majority of people struggling with

---

- Feelings of worthlessness or excessive guilt
- Diminished ability to think or concentrate, or indecisiveness
- Recurring thoughts of death or suicide

2. The symptoms must cause significant distress or impairment of social, occupational, or other important functions.

3. The symptoms do not result from another psychiatric diagnosis or a medical condition.

Within the category of major depression are various gradations of the illness—mild, moderate, severe without psychotic features, and severe with psychotic features. Not all forms of depression qualify as "major." Some syndromes have certain characteristics of depression but do not meet all of the criteria for a major depressive episode. Among them is dysthymic disorder, a low-grade depression of at least 2 years' duration. Subsyndromal depression is a mild form, but it does not have a specific time frame attached to it.

Source: American Psychiatric Association, Diagnostic and Statistical Manual of Mental Disorders, 4th ed. (Washington, DC: American Psychiatic Association, 1994).

depression. The bad news is that although some of the newer antidepressants have fewer side effects, they don't help all of the people all of the time. They may be effective for a while, only to stop working altogether.

The fact is, one-third of people diagnosed with depression do not respond to standard antidepressant therapy, and 20 to 30 percent stop taking their medications within a few weeks because of side effects. Of those who do respond to drug therapy, only about 25 to 30 percent achieve very good results. Even in this group, many are unable—or unwilling—to tolerate any adverse reactions for the long haul.[11] Mark, a 60-year-old physician, was just such a person.

Mark had experienced three episodes of major depression, each lasting about 6 months. Zoloft and Wellbutrin successfully wiped out his symptoms—along with his sexual function. He also complained of dry mouth, constipation, and mental fogginess.

After a couple of years, Mark decided that the antidepressants' side effects outweighed their benefits, and he slowly tapered off the medications. Although he wasn't as depressed as he had been before he'd begun drug therapy, he wasn't particularly happy or optimistic either. He described feeling "agitated and blue" at times. His patients and office staff complained that he seemed distracted.

At the suggestion of his psychiatrist, who had learned about *Rhodiola rosea* from Dick, Mark started taking the herb. He felt better almost immediately. Now on a daily maintenance dose of 500 milligrams, he says, "*Rhodiola rosea* stabilizes me. I have mood swings, but they're mild and appropriate to the situation. If I forget to take it for a couple of days, I feel worse again."

As part of his crusade to convince others that depression is nothing to be ashamed of, Mark frequently takes the herb in front of his patients. He even named his dog Rosavin.

A Blended Approach to Treatment

As psychiatrists, we treat people with all kinds of depression every day. Some who consult us already have tried a long list of antidepressants and, like Mark, are fed up with the side effects. Others feel that their symptoms have lifted somewhat, but they continue to describe their mood with words like "dull," "gray," and "colorless." They yearn for a little joie de vivre. In both cases, we've found that the most successful treatment regimen often combines prescription antidepressants with *Rhodiola rosea*.

Phyllis is a 44-year-old art therapist, wife, mother, and cancer survivor who suffered bouts of recurrent depression for many years. In the past, Prozac eased her symptoms, but it also caused insomnia and prevented her from having orgasms. She tried other antidepressants, but either they were of little help or they resulted in insomnia or overwhelming fatigue.

For Phyllis, the winning course of treatment turned out to be Effexor, a calming antidepressant, along with 600 milligrams a day of *Rhodiola rosea*. Despite serious setbacks, including a broken leg and the death of her father, she finally emerged from her depression, feeling more alert and energetic than ever. She even was able to sleep soundly through the night.

We've seen many other patients with depression get better while on antidepressants and not suffer terrible side effects. Still, they don't want to continue taking the pills indefinitely. Some are concerned about the long-term impact on their health; others favor natural substances whenever possible. Often in these cases, we find that the addition of *Rhodiola rosea* to the treatment regimen allows patients to gradually reduce, and sometimes taper off, prescription antidepressants with no ill effects.

Nan, a 55-year-old married attorney and mother of three, had a long history of dysthymia—chronic low-level depression and fatigue. She took Zoloft for 4 years, with good results. But the antidepressant affected her ability to have orgasms. This so distressed her that she avoided sexual intimacy with her husband, which resulted in problems in their marriage.

Dick advised Nan to take 300 milligrams of *Rhodiola rosea* daily, with the intent of helping her to gradually wean herself off Zoloft. Before long, she noticed dramatic improvement in her energy level and focus. She could accomplish much more at work and at home. As a bonus, she didn't get upset as easily. If something went wrong, she bounced back in no time.

Nan describes *Rhodiola rosea* as nothing short of a miracle. To her great delight, she was able to discontinue Zoloft 6 months after starting the herb and to enjoy sexual intimacy with her husband again.

Fatigue—whether mental, physical, or a combination of the two—is an almost universal feature of depression. Time and again, we have found that the powerful energy-boosting action of *Rhodiola rosea*—whether taken alone or with prescription antidepressants—goes a long way toward reinvigorating our patients' zest for life.

BIPOLAR DISORDER: STOPPING THE MOOD SWINGS

Steve is a 49-year-old museum curator with bipolar II disorder, the milder version of what was once called manic-depressive illness because of its characteristic pattern of mood swings. When he first came to see Dick, Steve was taking lithium, Tegretol (carbamazepine), Wellbutrin, and Zoloft to stabilize his mood. Most of the time, he felt grumpy and fatigued, and his libido wasn't as strong as it had been. He described "a feeling of paralysis" that prevented him from finishing his paperwork.

A daily 200-milligram dose of *Rhodiola rosea* recharged Steve's waning energy and freed him from his "paralysis." After 1 month on the herb, his mood swings stabilized, and his libido improved. In fact, he felt so energetic that he launched an exercise program. He was able to sustain a relationship, which eventually led to marriage.

As Steve says, "Once the rhodiola kicked in, it helped a lot. Today I feel good, active, engaged." And instead of four prescription medications, he takes just two, in addition to *Rhodiola rosea*.

Many people with bipolar disorder avoid treatment because they don't want to give up the excitement and euphoria—often expressed through high-risk behaviors such as reckless driving, overspending, and sexual promiscuity—that accompany their manic episodes. Fortunately, a growing class of medications called mood stabilizers—which include lithium, Tegretol, Depakote (divalproex), Lamictal (lamotrigine), and Trileptol (oxcarbazepine)—are so effective that many people with bipolar disorder who regularly take their medications can lead normal lives and do well in their careers. But sometimes, as in Steve's case, the drugs don't completely eliminate symptoms.

Any antidepressant or stimulant—whether it's a prescription pharmaceutical or an herbal preparation—has the potential to trigger a manic episode in someone with bipolar disorder. Generally, though, people who take mood stabilizers are at lower risk for this sort of reaction, especially if they have bipolar II. Those with bipolar I are prone to more severe—sometimes even suicidal—depression and more intense, agitated manic episodes. For this reason, doctors should monitor their treatment especially closely.

Because *Rhodiola rosea* has some stimulating action, it is not appropriate for bipolar patients whose mood swings are not stable. On the other hand, for someone whose mood swings are only moderate and who is taking mood stabilizers, *Rhodiola rosea* can be a valuable addition to treatment, under medical supervision.

ANXIETY:
A BY-PRODUCT OF STRESS

Does stress cause anxiety? Absolutely. Even if you don't have an anxiety disorder, you know that in certain stressful situations you feel nervous, worried, or perhaps fearful. No doubt you've experienced many of the bodily sensations that can accompany anxiety—a knot in your stomach, a lump in your throat, sweaty palms, rapid heartbeat, tightness in your chest, trembling, dizziness, or headache. More likely than not, though, you manage to calm yourself down.

Most of us find ways to cope with the stresses in our lives, or to avoid situations that create a sense of uneasiness. Episodes of extreme anxiety are blessedly brief and infrequent. But if they occur so often that they interfere with your capacity to function at work, at home, or in social situations, then you most likely have an anxiety disorder.

Patty, a 46-year-old recovering alcoholic and graphic designer, had been sober for 15 years. Still, she felt anxious much of the time—especially in social situations—and struggled to concentrate at work. What's more, she was having memory lapses, which fed into her fear that she might be suffering from early-onset Alzheimer's disease.

Like many recovering alcoholics, Patty was reluctant to try a prescription medication. But she was open to an alternative treatment.

When a colleague of ours suggested that she start with 100 milligrams of *Rhodiola rosea* a day and slowly increase her dosage to 300 milligrams a day, Patty agreed. The results were dramatic: Her anxiety subsided almost immediately, and 1 year later, she seldom if ever experienced anxious episodes—even at parties. She also noticed significant improvement in her concentration and memory.

Of course, people prone to depression may become anxious—or vice versa. Sometimes depression and anxiety go hand in hand.

Linda's life had been fraught with all kinds of emotional and psychological distress—a history of sexual abuse, separation anxiety, social anxiety, panic attacks, obsessive-compulsive symptoms, depression, anorexia, and substance abuse. By the time she got to Dick's office, she had tried a whole medicine chest full of drugs, including tricyclic antidepressants, Prozac, and Wellbutrin, among a score of others. Some of them eased her depression temporarily, but eventually they either stopped working or caused intolerable side effects.

More drugs were tried. So was phototherapy, with partial improvement. (Phototherapy involves the use of a special powerful light box.) At age 45, Linda was married, sober, and free from panic attacks and eating disorders. But she continued to feel depressed and anxious, especially at social gatherings with former drinking buddies.

Once Dick prescribed *Rhodiola rosea*, Linda's residual depression and social anxiety improved. But the herb really proved its worth 2 years later, the night Linda met up with her friends for a birthday bash. Before, a situation like that would have driven her to hide in the ladies' room for most of the evening, trembling and miserable. This time, to her surprise, she enjoyed herself immensely.

To this day, Linda continues to take 800 milligrams of *Rhodiola rosea* daily. In general, she is much calmer and more at ease with herself and others.

OBSESSIVE-COMPULSIVE DISORDER: WHEN THE MIND DOESN'T STOP

Most of us would admit to obsessive behavior at times. The object of our attention may be a love interest, a movie star, the NFL play-offs, even a box of Godiva chocolates. When we think about something over and over—without necessarily wanting to—we call it an obsession.

A compulsion, on the other hand, is when recurring thoughts drive us to repeat the same action for no real reason. Most compulsions are harmless. For instance, checking your e-mail 20 times a day—hoping for a message from that special someone—may be compulsive. But it won't hurt you.

People who are obsessive-compulsive tend to be good at taking care of details. But when these tendencies interfere with the ability to complete tasks or maintain satisfying relationships, a person may have bona fide obsessive-compulsive disorder, which can lead to job loss, social isolation, and depression.

By the time he turned 50, John had lost a number of jobs because he could never manage to finish his work. His missed deadlines were not a reflection of his intelligence; after all, he has a superior IQ. But no matter what he turned his attention to, he got stuck going over and over trivial details, never grasping the bigger picture. He hadn't paid his taxes for 10 years because he couldn't complete the forms.

John had tried numerous prescription medications for his severe obsessive-compulsive disorder, but none of them helped. In fact, he was nailed for several speeding tickets after one medication—Anafranil (clomipramine)—set off manic episodes.

To avoid inducing further mania, Dick treated John with a low dose of *Rhodiola rosea*—50 to 100 milligrams per day. Soon John was well enough to hold a management-level job and resume dating. In fact, if not for the herb, he says that he never would have been able to file his taxes.

Post-Traumatic Stress Disorder: History Repeats Itself

Post-traumatic stress disorder (PTSD) occurs after a traumatic event in which someone experiences or witnesses actual or threatened death or serious injury and feels intense fear, helplessness, or horror as a result. Long after the trauma, the person keeps reliving it in the form of recurring memories and images, dreams, and flashbacks. The person also has intense mental and physical reactions to anything that somehow evokes the original event. Between 10 and 30 percent of trauma survivors develop PTSD.

The amygdala and the hippocampus, both parts of the brain's limbic system, are responsible for processing fear reactions. Animal studies have shown that repeated stress can damage and destroy nerve cells in the hippocampus. The loss of nerve cells results in a loss of volume (size) of the hippocampus, which researchers can measure via magnetic resonance imaging (MRI).

Studies involving Vietnam War veterans, adult rape victims, and adult survivors of childhood physical and sexual abuse have shown that those who developed PTSD had smaller hippocampal volumes.[2, 3, 4] Not surprisingly, they also showed disturbances in the function of the hypothalamic-pituitary-adrenal axis, a component of the body's stress response system.

One possible reason that *Rhodiola rosea* could help people with PTSD—who are prone to depression, eating disorders, attention deficit disorder, and substance abuse—is that it calms the nervous system while protecting and energizing the nerves themselves. Still, this doesn't fully explain why the herb is such an effective treatment for PTSD. Perhaps when the central nervous system is more in balance, extreme reactions to triggering experiences or events are less likely to occur. And if there has been some damage to or disruption of neurotransmitter production in critical areas such as the hippocampal nerve cells, then *Rhodiola rosea* may help normalize the function of cells and increase the supply of neurotransmitters.

Tammy, a 37-year-old married woman, developed PTSD as a result of childhood sexual abuse. She also was plagued by periodic bouts of major depression. While a course of Zoloft partially lifted her mood, she continued to feel "flat and numb," and she lost all interest in sex.

When her doctor added 200 milligrams a day of *Rhodiola rosea* to her treatment regimen, Tammy's symptoms of depression and PTSD lessened significantly. But several months later, her depression—along with its characteristic low energy and low self-esteem—returned. When her doctor asked if she was doing anything differently, Tammy admitted that she had stopped taking *Rhodiola rosea*. She resumed treatment with the herb, and within a week her mood, energy, and focus improved markedly.

PTSD IN THE AFTERMATH OF WAR

The destruction, danger, and horror of war can traumatize soldiers and civilians alike. Sadly, given the confrontations and crises raging around the globe right now, this problem is not going away anytime soon.

The total breakdown of psychological defenses during warfare was referred to as shell shock during World War I. Today, you may hear it referred to as combat fatigue or combat stress reaction. Among Israeli soldiers who developed combat stress reaction during the

Lebanon War, 50 percent developed PTSD within 2 years. Another 19 percent who seemed to better tolerate combat conditions also developed PTSD within the same period.[9]

Although *Rhodiola rosea* helped our good friend Dr. Zakir Ramazanov endure the harsh physical conditions and extreme stress of serving in the Soviet army, he didn't discover the herb's most amazing benefits until after his discharge. By then he had begun suffering depression, flashbacks, and extreme emotional reactions—all classic symptoms of PTSD.

Zakir's story begins in Afghanistan. Like many college students in the former Soviet Union, he was not allowed to attend graduate school until he completed his military service. This is why, in 1979, he found himself in charge of a unit of soldiers fighting in the rugged mountains of Afghanistan.

During the winter of 1980, his comrade Sergei—like many of the soldiers—received a holiday box from home. While most of the boxes overflowed with beautiful fruits and other treats, Sergei's contained a bunch of ugly roots. "What the hell is that?" Zakir remembers asking his friend, who was from Siberia. "He told me that it was a medicinal root called *Rhodiola rosea*, and that I would appreciate it later. Even though it was ugly, the cut root smelled like a rose. And it made a wonderful tea."

Zakir—a large, strong man who had played professional soccer—noticed that the soldiers who drank the tea were better able to hike through deep snow over high mountain passes, carrying full gear, AK-47s, and gas masks. And they did it on 4 hours of sleep a night. So Zakir decided to try *Rhodiola rosea* for himself. "Once I started drinking the tea, I woke up without the usual soreness in my muscles, and I recovered much faster after each mission," he recalls. "But then I left the army, and I forgot all about it."

A few years later, Zakir was working for the Soviet Institute of Energy, designing solar batteries for the *Mir* space station—a good job with an excellent salary. But instead of enjoying his success, he developed severe stress symptoms and became depressed for the first time in his life. Determined to understand what was happening to him, Zakir read as many books as he could find on PTSD in Vietnam veterans. He discovered that the symptoms can occur long after the stressful events have passed. That's when he began to put together the pieces of his own illness.

"I saw so many people killed in the army," Zakir says now. "We couldn't even react to it because if you cry in that situation, you get killed. It's self-preservation. You must mobilize every emotional and physical resource just to survive. But then when it's over and you expect to be happy, the stress comes rushing back. I couldn't sleep. I was very emotional. I didn't want to see anything, even a cow or a chicken, get killed. My skin would crawl with goose bumps.

"I tried everything, from sedatives to herbs. None of it worked. My mood constantly fluctuated—good, bad, up, down. Things that normally would have excited me instead fell flat.

"Then I heard a lecture on *Rhodiola rosea*, and I remembered Sergei's tea. I became obsessed with learning more about the herb. Fortunately for me, in 1984 I received an invitation to present a lecture in Siberia, where *Rhodiola rosea* grows wild. When I saw it, it was like love at first sight.

"I took some home with me and began using it right away. Its effects were even stronger than before. Within a month, the terrible post-traumatic stress symptoms were gone. I had more energy during the day, and I could sleep at night.

"After about 2 months, the depression went away completely. By then I no longer was overreacting to things, as the images of war had stopped running through my head. I became tremendously productive in my work, publishing 10 scientific papers in 1 year and receiving many academic honors and research opportunities. In fact, I first came to the United States on an invitation from the National Academy of Sciences."

Since his recovery from PTSD with help from *Rhodiola rosea*, Zakir has dedicated himself to protecting the plants from overharvesting. He also is committed to maintaining the purity of the root extracts, and he's experimenting with raising the herb hydroponically. The seedlings are planted in different locations around the world so mankind always will have a supply. As Zakir says, "I want others with physical or mental stress to be able to get well, as I did."

❧❧❧

How to take Rhodiola rosea . . .

FOR DEPRESSION, ANXIETY, AND OTHER MOOD DISORDERS

If you're taking prescription antidepressants, mood stabilizers, or anti-anxiety medication, be sure to consult your doctor before trying Rhodiola rosea. *If your doctor is not familiar with the herb, you can lend him your book. Or you can direct him to the American Botanical Council's* HerbalGram *Web site (www.herbalgram.org), where he can download a copy of our article* "Rhodiola rosea: A Phytomedicinal Overview," *which appeared in the fall 2002 issue of* HerbalGram *magazine.*

The amount of Rhodiola rosea *that you need will depend on your size, your individual body chemistry, and the sensitivity of your nervous system. In general, your best bet is to start with one 100-milligram capsule ½ hour before breakfast, on an empty stomach. If after 3 days you show no signs of overstimulation or other adverse effects, you can take a second 100-milligram capsule ½ hour before lunch.*

Wait 3 to 7 days to see how you feel. Many people notice improvement within a week, even on a modest dose. If you need more, add a second capsule ½ hour before breakfast. After another 3 to 7 days, you can add a second capsule ½ hour before lunch, for a total of four capsules—or 400 milligrams—a day. Allow at least 2 weeks at this dosage to see results.

Most people don't need to go higher than 400 milligrams of Rhodiola rosea *a day. If by chance you do, try a third capsule before breakfast, as long as you don't feel agitated or have trouble sleeping. Wait 2 more weeks, then, if necessary, take a third capsule before lunch, for a total of six capsules—600 milligrams—per day.*

CHAPTER 10

Fight Back
AGAINST
FATIGUE

Everywhere we turn, friends, patients, and colleagues seem to be feeling burned-out, overwhelmed, fried. "Too much to do, not enough energy" is their standard refrain.

Though in most cases it isn't a diagnosable disease with abnormalities that can be detected in the lab, exhaustion is looking more and more like *the* modern pandemic among otherwise healthy people. This state of affairs is reflected in doctor visits: A 2003 survey of general practitioners revealed that one in seven working people who scheduled office appointments did so because of fatigue.[1]

As a group, women seem to be the hardest hit. This makes sense when you consider that over the past few decades, they have taken on more roles than ever before. Currently, 73 percent of all women with school-age children work outside the home.

This is not to imply that men aren't feeling exhausted in record numbers. They, too, are subject to the multiple pressures of living in a fiercely competitive, wired society. The difference is that women are taking on demanding jobs—often positions with greater responsibilities—while still serving as chief cook, bottle washer, and nurturer on the home front. The result is a high-stress balancing act, too often without a safety net below.

Evidently, the problem is global. In a recent survey of women public health employees in Sweden, between 26 and 34 percent reported job-related emotional exhaustion. Many also complained of fatigue, sleep disturbances, and cognitive impairment.[7] Here in the United States, a 2003 survey of people living in Wichita, Kansas, found that 373 women per 100,000 had been diagnosed with chronic fatigue syndrome, compared with 83 men per 100,000.[8]

Ann is the perfect example of a working woman who was losing ground in the battle to keep up with the demands of her busy life.

When she first came to see Pat, Ann—a 40-year-old office manager and divorced mother of three—reported that she had been feeling more and more fatigued over the course of several months. Recently, the situation had taken a turn for the worse: She had developed four upper respiratory infections, a runaway appetite that resulted in a weight gain of 25 pounds, insomnia, and irritability that seemed to intensify by the day. She also had experienced joint pain, muscle weakness, and dizzy spells every time she tried exercising.

Ann's professional life was going downhill, too. Many days she either called in sick or left work early. Now she not only felt sick and exhausted, but she was also afraid of losing her job.

As soon as Ann began telling her story, Pat realized that no matter what else might be going on clinically, Ann's energy reserves had dipped extremely low. At the same time, her stress level probably had never been higher. She was trapped in a vicious cycle that was threatening to spiral out of control: The sicker she got, the less able she was to meet her obligations, and the more panicky she felt. At night, instead of replenishing her dwindling energy reserves with a good night's sleep, she would lie awake, frightened and worried that she wouldn't have the strength to get through the next day.

During their first meeting, Pat asked Ann to consider her many responsibilities and to figure out which ones were ironclad and which could be tabled until further notice. For example, she needed to feed her children, but she certainly didn't need to make every meal from scratch. Nor did she need to drive several miles out of her way to take them to school every morning, making her own commute 45 minutes longer. The school bus would do just fine.

Ann quickly understood that she wasn't simply trying to be a good parent. She was compensating for the painful divorce that essentially had left her children fatherless. She also recognized that if she didn't make her health a priority, the entire family would suffer. She was surprised and relieved to discover that many of the tasks she previously had considered do-or-die could be postponed or eliminated altogether.

Next, Pat prescribed a course of *Rhodiola rosea*—100 milligrams three times a day—to help Ann recoup her energy. Almost immediately, she was sleeping better. Within a week, she noticed improvement in her mood. For the first time in months, she was able to calmly negotiate how much time her son could spend playing his computer games, instead of flying off the handle as soon as he sat down in front of the screen.

Over the next few weeks, Ann's appetite returned to normal, and she was able to resume her daily power walk. The extra pounds gradually melted away, and the joint pain, muscle weakness, and dizzy spells completely disappeared.

Today Ann is working full-time once again. She continues to actively seek out new opportunities to enjoy both the riches of her family life and the rewards of her career—*without* sacrificing herself or her health in the process.

THE MANY FACES OF FATIGUE

The word *fatigue* describes a broad spectrum of complaints—from moderate everyday tiredness, to the sort of exhaustion or burnout that plagued Ann, to severe chronic fatigue syndrome. The causes of fatigue can be difficult to tease apart because often more than one is to blame. For example, fatigue could be a symptom of medical illness, a sign of psychological distress, the aftermath of an infection—or a combination of all three. And then there is mental fatigue—the fuzzy thinking and impaired concentration that can result from overwork, stress, or aging.

The fact is, nearly everyone—even those in excellent health—experiences bouts of fatigue at certain points in their lives. Because doctors often struggle to pinpoint the source of the problem, patients may be put through an endless battery of tests, only to end up with no conclusive diagnosis. Just as often, they're on the receiving end of a long series of ineffectual treatments that leave them feeling hopeless. Rosemary, a 51-year-old freelance journalist, fell into this category.

When Rosemary met Dick, the first words out of her mouth were "I really don't know why I'm here. I've been to internists, shrinks, nutritionists, acupuncturists, chiropractors, homeopaths—you name it. One doctor told me that I have chronic fatigue syndrome; another said that it's fibromyalgia. But no matter what treatment they prescribed, I still felt so wiped out that I couldn't think straight. I'd say that you are my last hope, only I don't have much hope left."

Dick told Rosemary that since her lab tests were within the normal range—as they had been all along—isolating the exact cause of her chronic exhaustion probably would be next to impossible. Even so, Dick had a hunch that *Rhodiola rosea* would help restore her physical and mental energy. Rosemary was skeptical, but she agreed to try the herb for 2 months. After just 1 month, she reported that she had been able to finish writing an article that was long overdue. By the next month, she described feeling like her "old self" for the first time in more than 2 years.

Rosemary continues to take 200 milligrams of *Rhodiola rosea* twice each day, before breakfast and before lunch. Now she's thinking about applying for a full-time editorial position, something she never would have considered just a few months earlier.

NEURASTHENIA: A DISORDER BY MANY OTHER NAMES

In 1869, George Beard coined the term *neurasthenia* to describe a chronic functional disease of the nervous system, characterized by weakness and fatigue. He attributed these symptoms to the increased mental and physical stress of urbanization and the industrial revolution. The diagnosis caught on like wildfire, especially in the Orient and Europe. It became fashionable for members of the upper and middle classes to rejuvenate their exhausted nervous systems at health spas.

In 1979, the American Psychiatric Association deemed *neurasthenia* too vague. In a departure from the World Health Organization, the APA decided to drop the term from the third edition of the *Diagnostic and Statistical Manual of Mental Disorders* (DSM-III, 1979).[6] That's why people like Rosemary, who once might have been diagnosed with neurasthenia, now are told that they suffer from chronic fatigue syndrome or fibromyalgia—diagnoses that can be just as vague and difficult to establish with certainty. Sometimes the source of persistent fatigue is subsyndromal or low-level depression, which frequently goes undiagnosed.

No matter what its name, the condition once known as neurasthenia is widespread. In fact, in many other countries, it still is a viable diagnosis. The World Health Organization, in its book *International Classification of Diseases*, describes neurasthenia as a condition not caused by a mental or emotional disorder and characterized by:

- Persistent and distressing feelings of either exhaustion after minor mental effort or fatigue after minor physical effort

- An inability to recover through rest, relaxation, or enjoyment

- One or more symptoms such as muscle aches or pains, tension headaches, dizziness, sleep disturbances, irritability, or an inability to relax

In the Soviet Union in the 1970s and 1980s, patients with symptoms of neurasthenia—including fatigue, insomnia, decline in work capacity, headache, poor appetite, irritability, and neuroses—participated in clinical trials involving *Rhodiola rosea*. Although the research designs and diagnostic categories do not meet all modern scientific standards, they do provide valuable clinical observations. For example, more than 400 patients with neurasthenic symptoms improved on a low dose of *Rhodiola rosea*—just 150 milligrams a day—over a period ranging from 10 days to 4 months.[9]

WHEN STRESS ENTERS THE PICTURE

For some people, bouts of extreme fatigue are intermittent and time-limited, and the cause is anything but mysterious. In these cases, there is an obvious stressor, and the fatigue usually fades along with the source of stress—which can run the gamut from a sudden loss or serious illness to a high-pressure work situation. Jim, a 50-year-old business executive and one of Dick's patients, offers a good example of this type of fatigue.

Jim's workload comes in periodic bursts. Although his baseline work pace is a reasonable 40 hours a week, three or four times a year he attends international conferences that require him to travel back and forth across several time zones. This goes on for about a month. During these periods, Jim works 20-hour days under intense pressure.

The combination of job stress, sleep deprivation, and jet lag had been taking a growing toll. Exhausted and bleary-eyed, Jim was struggling to continually perform at the high level expected of him. Then, during the third week of an overseas business trip, he developed a nasty sore throat. Dick prescribed *Rhodiola rosea*, and Jim immediately took his first 450-milligram dose. The following morning, his sore throat was much better. As a bonus, he felt more energized than usual.

Over the next month, Jim noticed that the herb had replenished his energy reserves. He could work long hours fruitfully, with almost no effects from jet lag.

DEPRESSION AS CAUSE AND EFFECT

It's a little bit like the chicken-or-egg question: Which comes first, fatigue or depression? Actually, it works both ways. Chronic fatigue and pain can cause depression. Conversely, depression and excessive stress can trigger fatigue and physical symptoms, including pain. This creates a dilemma for doctors: Should they treat chronic fatigue as a medical or a psychological disorder? Of course, in an ideal world, they would treat the whole person by addressing both physical and emotional symptoms, regardless of the source. But this doesn't always happen.

Delia, a 39-year-old physician, is like many people who consult us because their doctors have not been able to determine whether their fatigue is driving their depression, or vice versa. Often they already have tried treatment with antidepressants and other conventional drug therapies, without much success.

When she first met Dick, Delia was struggling with severe fatigue and trying to keep up with her medical practice. She was feeling so worn-out that she had given up her daily gym workouts, which only worsened her depression. What's more, she had been taking three different antibiotics and heavy-duty steroids to clear up her recurrent sinusitis. Unfortunately, she didn't feel any better.

One day, desperate to break the downward spiral, Delia headed out for a run, only to collapse. She went to see numerous specialists, who told her that she had tender "trigger points," a symptom of chronic fatigue syndrome and fibromyalgia. After that, even a short walk would land her in bed for days.

As she became weaker, Delia felt increasingly worried and hopeless. One of her doctors prescribed a series of antidepressants, but they left her feeling either too jittery or overly sedated. Finally, on the verge of giving up the medical practice that she loved, she made an appointment to see Dick. He suggested a course of *Rhodiola rosea*—300 milligrams a day.

Within a few weeks, Delia was showing signs of improvement. After 2 months, she was completely free of fatigue and depression and feeling well enough to resume her daily workouts. Although many of our patients find that they do best when they stay on *Rhodiola rosea* for the long term, Delia was so much better that she decided to stop taking the herb. She has been well ever since.

THE INFECTION CONNECTION

While studying people who showed signs of neurasthenia, Soviet researchers determined that many of them first developed symptoms following an infection, such as influenza. We, too, have seen numerous patients who experienced extreme physical and/or mental fatigue following treatment for various infections, including Lyme disease.

Even when antibiotics presumably have cleared away the active infection, residual symptoms may persist for months or even years. Besides general fatigue, these symptoms can include fuzzy thinking, difficulty concentrating, impaired memory, insomnia, headache, muscle and tendon pain, weakness, and neuralgia—a poorly understood type of pain that originates in nerve endings.

Like Delia, many of our patients already have consulted doctor after doctor by the time they make an appointment with us. They worry that their symptoms are "all in their heads." The lack of abnormal laboratory or radiology findings—not to mention the absence of a viable treatment—further fuels their self-doubt.

As we saw in Delia's case, the prospect of endless fatigue, pain, and impaired function can lead to depression and anxiety. Though some doctors accurately diagnose depression, few recognize that it may be secondary to the residual symptoms, not the other way around.

As time passes and their health deteriorates further, desperate patients try almost any treatment that they can find. Some ask their dentists to remove their mercury fillings. Others invest in "adrenal support" supplements. Jeanne is one patient who had been through many traditional and alternative treatments before scheduling an appointment with Pat.

Jeanne always had been an active, energetic woman. In addition to raising five children, she enjoyed tending a houseful of animals as well as her extensive gardens. As her kids grew up and started families of their own, Jeanne's farm continued to be the center of their activity. She was blessed with excellent health and many creative and fulfilling interests.

Then, at age 68, Jeanne was bitten by a deer tick. Her doctor prescribed a 2-week course of antibiotics—an inadequate treatment. Over the next 7 years, she developed joint pain, fatigue, heat intolerance, anxiety, and eventually an irregular heartbeat.

Jeanne sought the advice of a specialist, who diagnosed residual symptoms of Lyme disease. The doctor gave Jeanne another course of antibiotics and put her on heart medication. Still, she found that even minimal exertion would trigger an irregular heartbeat. This only added to her anxiety. Discouraged about her health and unable to enjoy her usual activities, she sank into depression.

Jeanne returned to her doctor, who prescribed an even stronger antibiotic. It cured her joint pain, but her nervous system did not recover. She remained weak, nervous, depressed, off balance, and mentally dull. She took medication for anxiety, as well as dozens of supplements and low-dose cortisol for "adrenal burnout." She even tried replacing her dental fillings to avoid contamination by "mercury toxicity"—all to no avail.

Ten years after her tick bite, Jeanne finally came to see Pat. She was upset, tearful, and frightened. Her life had spun out of control, and nothing seemed able to bring it back on track.

Because Jeanne's system had become extremely reactive to medication, antidepressants were out of the question. Instead, Pat started her on a tiny dose of *Rhodiola rosea*—just one-sixth of a 100-milligram capsule every morning. Miraculously, she showed improvement on the very first day she took the herb. She said that she felt mentally alert, with her mind "clicking the way it used to." An energy surge inspired her to go for an afternoon walk in the hills, where she noticed greater strength in her leg muscles. At the end of the day, she realized that for the first time in months, she hadn't even thought about taking an anti-anxiety pill.

Over the next few days, Jeanne's energy level continued to rise, but the herb began to upset her stomach. When she stopped her treatment for 2 days, her mind seemed to slow down almost immediately. Fortunately, taking ginger capsules ½ hour prior to her dose of *Rhodiola rosea* calmed her upset stomach, so she was able to resume her treatment.

Jeanne's optimal dosage of *Rhodiola rosea* turned out to be one-half of a capsule before breakfast, and again before lunch. By the third week, she felt like a new person—or, rather, the person she had been before her illness.

Of course, post-Lyme infection doesn't always respond so dramatically to such small doses of *Rhodiola rosea*. But with larger doses— usually 200 to 300 milligrams twice daily—symptoms often get better over time. In cases of long-standing illness, certain symptoms may not show improvement for several months. Yet remarkably, for many of the patients who have come to us for help with residual symptoms, *Rhodiola rosea* is the only treatment to produce results.

A WORD ABOUT ADRENAL BURNOUT

If you're feeling stressed-out and exhausted, you may be wondering if you're suffering from adrenal burnout. The answer is: probably not.

Adrenal burnout is a catchy phrase that convinces people to buy adrenal support supplements. As a medical diagnosis, it has no scientific basis. As you've seen in this chapter, people who say they feel "burned-out" may be suffering from neurasthenia, depression, stress, or an underlying medical condition. But there simply is no evidence that the adrenal glands stop functioning because of stress.

When something triggers the body's stress response, the adrenals—which rest atop the kidneys and are components of the hypothalamic-pituitary-adrenal axis (HPA)—release the hormone cortisol. Researchers have determined that most people who describe themselves as "burned-out" actually have the same cortisol levels and stress responses as people who are healthy.

Nevertheless, in a few studies, some participants with "burnout" did show higher-than-usual cortisol levels during the first hour after waking up in the morning.[4] Then levels returned to normal and stayed there the rest of the day. Even among people with chronic fatigue syndrome, only 30 percent showed a brief elevation in cortisol first thing in the morning. In the remaining 70 percent, levels of the hormone held steady.

The jump in cortisol that occurs during the first hour after awakening indicates an imbalance in the regulatory feedback systems of the HPA axis. It is not a sign of a shortage of cortisol or of any abnormality in the adrenal glands.

This helps explain why attempts to treat burnout or chronic fatigue with cortisol supplementation, in the form of hydrocortisone, have had mixed or weak results.[3] In one recent study, which involved 100 patients with chronic fatigue syndrome, 50 received low-dose hydrocortisone, while the rest took a placebo. By the end of the study, which lasted 6 months, the research found no measurable difference in fatigue or well-being between the two groups.[2]

According to other studies, the drop in cortisol levels that occurs in some people with chronic fatigue syndrome is due to an imbalance at the higher levels of the HPA feedback system—that is, in the pituitary gland and hypothalamus—rather than in the adrenals. In these people, adrenal capacity appears to be normal.[5]

The false notion that stress can exhaust the adrenal glands, causing a cortisol deficiency that's correctable with supplements, has been exploited to sell useless products. Unfortunately, it also has led consumers suffering from fatigue to overlook other treatments, like *Rhodiola rosea*, that are proven to replenish energy reserves.

Please note that adrenal burnout is different from adrenal insufficiency, a serious autoimmune disease that usually results from inflammation of the adrenal glands or a disease of the pituitary gland. This leads to a severe decline in the release of glucocorticoids such as cortisol. Symptoms of adrenal insufficiency include fatigue, weight loss, and anorexia. If left untreated, the disease can be fatal. Thankfully, though, it is quite rare.

❦

How to take Rhodiola rosea . . .

To Combat Fatigue

As with any treatment, we suggest starting with a small amount of Rhodiola rosea *and gradually increasing your dosage. Doing this not only allows your system to adjust, it also enables you to monitor the herb's effectiveness.*

For symptoms of fatigue, we recommend an initial dose of 100 milligrams of Rhodiola rosea, *taken ½ hour before breakfast on an empty stomach. If after 3 to 7 days you're tolerating this amount well, you can add a 100-milligram capsule ½ hour before lunch. Some people will need as many as two capsules twice a day, while others may feel overstimulated with just one capsule. If this happens to you, you can reduce your dose by opening a capsule and pouring a fraction of the contents into tea or juice. Reseal the capsule and use the remainder the next day.*

CHAPTER 11

E n h a n c e   Y o u r

SEXUAL

VITALITY

Sexual pleasure deepens the sense of connectedness between two people. But its shadow side—sexual dysfunction—has the opposite effect, driving a wedge into intimate relationships. Struggles with desire and performance can fuel disappointment, frustration, anger, depression, anxiety, and poor self-esteem in one or both partners.

Although our society encourages frank discussion of all aspects of sexuality, many of us feel too embarrassed or ashamed to seek help for our sexual problems. The media's idealized and misleading images of great sex only worsen our feelings of inadequacy. But we don't get to see our idols of the big and small screens after a long day in the studio. Just like the rest of us, when they go home feeling stressed and drained, they are *not* in the mood for love. And they can't always perform in bed, either.

For both women and men, sexual dysfunction often takes one of three forms: low libido—that is, lack of sexual desire—or difficulty achieving arousal or orgasm. Pinpointing the source of the problem can be a challenge for doctors and patients alike. This is because so many variables come into play—including age, diet, lifestyle, stress level, medical conditions and medications, emotional issues, cultural attitudes, and past experiences, to highlight just some of the possibilities.

WOMEN, MEN, AND SEX

An estimated 30 to 50 percent of adult women—a daunting number—report some sort of sexual dysfunction. The most common complaint is lack of sexual desire. In an Internet survey of healthy women—the majority of whom were married and premenopausal—77 percent reported low libido, while 62 percent had difficulty with arousal, and 56 percent with orgasm. More than half of these women considered seeking help, but most were resigned to toughing it out on their own.[5]

The perception of low libido as a sexual problem is a relatively modern phenomenon. Not so long ago, in Victorian times, the absence of sexual desire was considered a virtue. This is hardly the case in the sex-crazed culture of today.

While men also experience diminished interest in sex, for them the most common sexual problem is erectile dysfunction (ED)—the inability to sustain an erection through orgasm. ED affects 30 to 50 percent of men worldwide, including about 30 million in the United States alone.[17] Numerous factors can increase the risk of ED, including age, other medical conditions, certain medications, stress, and depression.

Interestingly, one of the chief contributors to ED may be lack of exercise. The condition is less likely to occur in men who are physically active at work or during their leisure hours.[14, 20]

Despite the availability of effective treatments, only 20 percent of men who struggle with ED ever seek medical help.[7] For those who do, Viagra (sildenafil) usually is the treatment of choice.

THE LITTLE BLUE PILL VERSUS
THE CENTURIES-OLD HERB

Viagra was the first in a new class of medications called phosphodi-esterase-5 inhibitors, which may turn the tide in erectile dysfunction. In studies, about 57 percent of men with ED who tried Viagra reported successful intercourse, compared with just 21 percent of those taking a placebo. The drug also may prolong erection in men prone to premature ejaculation.

While the side effects of Viagra tend to be mild,[11] men with coronary artery disease should proceed with caution. In general, the drug is considered safe as long as it is not taken within 24 hours of nitrate medications, which are used to alleviate angina. The combination of Viagra and nitrates can be fatal, causing heart attack and sudden death.[23]

More recent additions to the phosphodiesterase-5 inhibitors include Levitra (vardenafil) and Cialis (tadalafil), both of which have proven effective in treating many cases of ED. In fact, they're said to last longer than Viagra, though no comparison studies have been done to date. In general, the side effects of Levitra and Cialis are mild and may include headache, flushing, stomach upset, and transient changes in color perception. As with Viagra, these newer medications should never be taken too closely to nitrates. In fact, the time between doses may need to be even longer than 24 hours, since Levitra and Cialis linger in the body.

For decades, most pharmaceutical research of sexual dysfunction focused on men, with Viagra as the result. Lately, however, sexual dysfunction in women has been attracting more attention. While Viagra is not the breakthrough treatment for women that it has been for men, it can help women achieve sexual arousal and orgasm when—

and *only* when—the sexual dysfunction results from some other medication, such as an antidepressant.[15, 16] Unfortunately, in a study involving hundreds of women with low libido, participants did not notice any increase in sexual responsiveness when they took Viagra.[4]

Still, considering that the "little blue pill" is safe and effective for men, as well as for women with medication-induced sexual dysfunction, you may wonder why anyone would want to take anything else. There are several reasons. First, if 57 percent of men with erectile dysfunction who try Viagra get results from it, that leaves the other 43 percent out in the cold. Second, some don't like the side effects, which can include sinus congestion, headache, flushing, stomach upset, and visual disturbances.

Third, even for those who benefit from the drug and can tolerate the side effects, Viagra is not cheap. At $9 to $11 per tablet, twice-weekly use costs about $80 a month. If just 70 percent of the 30 million American men with erectile dysfunction were to take Viagra once a week, the national cost would be $210 million a week—which probably would send insurance premiums through the roof!

Even so, perhaps the most compelling reason to contemplate alternatives to Viagra is that the drug does absolutely nothing to boost sexual desire in men or women—a benefit that our favorite herb, *Rhodiola rosea*, is known for throughout Russia, Siberia, and other parts of Asia. What's more, while it isn't as potent as Viagra for erectile dysfunction, *Rhodiola rosea* definitely can help. Doctors in Siberia and the Republic of Georgia regularly prescribe a tincture of the root extract to improve sexual function in men.

At age 40, Sandy, an unmarried office manager, wasn't interested in sex. In fact, she had lost her libido sometime around her thirtieth birthday. She had been on and off antidepressants since then. Even during the "off" periods, she felt no desire for sex.

While on Zoloft, Sandy decided to experiment with 400 milligrams of *Rhodiola rosea* a day. Almost immediately, she felt sexually alive again. Her head swirled with romantic and erotic fantasies, so much so that no matter where she was—at home, at work, or in line at the supermarket—she couldn't help but think about sex.

This state of hyperarousal proved a little too intense for Sandy. She told her doctor that she was having trouble with "Love Potion #9." He cut her dosage in half, to 200 milligrams a day—which turned out to be just right.

DEPRESSION AND SEXUAL DYSFUNCTION

More than 70 percent of patients with major depression (see page 134 for a description) report sexual dysfunction.[10] Unfortunately, the "cure" for depression can be as bad as the condition itself. Antidepressant medications, particularly selective serotonin reuptake inhibitors such as Prozac and Zoloft, are a major cause of sexual problems.

Given a choice between being depressed and having a satisfying sex life, many patients feel caught between a rock and a hard place. Time and again, we have found that treatment with *Rhodiola rosea* can make all the difference because the herb improves both sexual function and mood. What's more, it's the only sex enhancer we know that revives *both* male and female libidos. Patrick and Angela are good examples.

Prone to depression, Patrick had tried many antidepressants over the years. By the time he turned 50, both he and his wife were frustrated by his irritable mood, constant fatigue, and lack of sexual desire. Dick suggested a daily course of 200 milligrams of *Rhodiola rosea*. Within 4 weeks, Patrick was a changed man. His mood and energy had improved, and best of all, his long-lost libido had returned.

In many ways, Angela was Patrick's female counterpart. A 42-year-old married sales manager and mother of two, she was typical of women whose once-strong libidos feel like ancient history. Although she was depressed, she was determined to do something about her predicament—something, that is, besides taking antidepressants. She had tried them in the past but couldn't tolerate the side effects.

Angela consulted a nurse-practitioner, who recommended 300 milligrams a day of *Rhodiola rosea*. Within 1 month, she felt 10 years younger and much happier, with energy to spare. And after her years of being exiled in a "sexual wasteland," her desire for sex returned full force.

Of course, the question often arises: Does depression cause sexual dysfunction, or is it the other way around? The answer, not surprisingly, is that their relationship is a two-way street. Depression is a risk factor for sexual dysfunction, and vice versa.[19]

For men, the situation gets even more complicated once heart disease steps in. So many studies have linked depression, erectile dysfunction, and coronary artery disease that doctors now use the abbreviation DEC to describe this common constellation of problems.[22] Dan, a 60-year-old businessman, is among the growing number of men who've received the triple whammy DEC diagnosis.

When Dan first came to see Dick, antidepressant medications had all but wiped out his sex drive, and his blood pressure had become unstable. Dick recommended *Rhodiola rosea*, 100 milligrams a day. Fortunately, Dan had a triple whammy response to the herb: His mood and cardiovascular function—as indicated by his exercise tolerance—improved noticeably, as did his sexual performance.

THE EFFECTS OF "THE CHANGE"

With the onset of menopause, many women develop sexual problems as a result of physiological changes that also have psychological and societal implications. For example, the decline in estrogen and progesterone characteristic of menopause contributes to loss of muscle mass and skin firmness, as well as wrinkles, thinning hair, and changes in body shape. In a culture that uses youthful beauty as the measure of female attractiveness, a menopausal woman may become insecure about her femininity and sexuality. At the same time, reduced hormone levels can result in vaginal dryness, leading to painful intercourse and loss of libido.

Treatment for sexual dysfunction during menopause is most effective when it addresses the full spectrum of changes triggered by the decline in estrogen and progesterone—from physical discomforts, to emotional and cognitive symptoms, to relationship issues. Some women become especially vulnerable to sociocultural pressures at this time in their lives. They may need extra support from family and friends to overcome negative attitudes toward aging and to keep the onset of menopause from undermining their sense of self-worth and their essential feminine identity.

For relief from the physical discomforts of menopause, particularly vaginal dryness and hot flashes, many women once turned to hormone replacement therapy (HRT). But recent findings about the health risks associated with HRT have made it a far less appealing solution.

Like estrogen and progesterone, testosterone—a hormone produced by the ovaries—declines with the approach of menopause. (That's right: Testosterone is not just a "male" hormone.) It also may be a factor in the loss of sexual desire and response. Dehydroepiandrosterone (DHEA), a testosterone precursor released by the adrenal cortex, may help normalize testosterone levels. But an autoimmune disease called adrenal insufficiency can deplete DHEA, too. In one study of women with documented adrenal insufficiency and low DHEA, those who took DHEA supplements felt less fatigue, stronger libido, and greater sexual satisfaction than those who took a placebo.[3]

Only women with confirmed testosterone or DHEA deficiency, as measured by a blood test, should try DHEA supplementation—and then only with medical supervision. Their doctors can ensure that they're taking a good-quality preparation and can closely monitor their testosterone levels. One word of caution: In rare cases, some DHEA may convert to a form of estrogen called estradiol, which could increase the risk of breast, uterine, or ovarian cancer in post-menopausal women.[6]

Marian, a 52-year-old musician, complained of low energy as well as lack of libido and orgasms as she entered menopause. When Dick tested her DHEA level, it was low. Supplementation replenished her DHEA supply, which had a positive effect on her energy and mood—but not on her sexual responsiveness. Once she added 300 milligrams a day of *Rhodiola rosea* to her regimen, Marian happily recovered her sexual desire and her capacity for sexual pleasure.

The impact of hormones on female sexuality is not well understood. So far, the results of scientific studies have been inconsistent. Replacing estrogen, progesterone, and/or testosterone has improved sexual function in only a minority of menopausal women who've tried it. Perhaps this is because so many other factors influence female sexuality, including the quality of intimacy, the potency of fantasies, and the highly subjective concepts of love and satisfaction—all of which defy measurement.

FROM RUSSIA WITH LOVE

As far as we know, *Rhodiola rosea* is the only treatment that can enhance sexual desire, arousal, and the capacity for orgasm in women, as well as heighten sex drive in men—all without any serious side effects. The Russians have been in on this well-kept secret for centuries. Traditionally, in the mountain villages of the Caucasus and Altai mountain ranges of Siberia, new brides receive a large bouquet of mature *Rhodiola rosea* roots to ensure fertility and the birth of healthy children. Older villagers rely on the herb to preserve their sex drive and sexual satisfaction. Physicians and healers routinely recommend it as well.

Clinical research has confirmed the benefits of *Rhodiola rosea* for men. In a small study involving 35 men with erectile dysfunction and/or premature ejaculation, taking 100 milligrams *Rhodiola rosea* every day for 3 months improved sexual performance in 74 percent of the participants. It also raised 17-ketosteroids to normal levels and increased the number of lecithin globules (liposomes) in semen.[18] Why are these changes important?

When glucocorticoids from the adrenal glands and androgens from the testes get broken down or metabolized, among the by-products are 17-ketosteroids. So doctors can measure the 17-ketosteroids to evaluate both adrenal function and fertility. Some 17-ketosteroids, such as DHEA and DHEAS (dehydroepiandrosterone sulfate), have anti-inflammatory and antioxidant properties as well.[13]

The rise in the amount of lecithin in semen is good news for sperm cells. During their production and development, these cells—which carry our genetic code—are very vulnerable to damage. Excessive heat, cold, radiation, or chemical toxins can disrupt delicate chromosomes, especially when they are replicating rapidly. Animal breeders have learned that by storing sperm in solutions made with lecithin—found in egg yolks—they can protect the cells from damage during cold storage or freezing and increase the rate of successful inseminations. Semen that's protected by lecithin is less likely to contain abnormal sperm forms.[1, 12]

DRAGGING THEIR TAILS
BEHIND THEM

In a recent issue of the journal *Advanced Experiments in Medical Biology*, we noticed an article with the alarming title "The Human Spermatozoon—Not Waving But Drowning." According to the article, humans have the poorest-quality semen of all mammalian species. What surprised us most is that the semen of "normal," fertile men can carry up to 85 percent abnormal sperm. The consequences are low fertility in men, as well as spontaneous miscarriages in women and a variety of cancers and birth defects in children.[2]

In the past, doctors routinely attributed early miscarriage to what they describe as "blighted ovum," or an egg with defective DNA. Now it appears that the DNA in the sperm may be to blame as well. Sometimes sperm cell abnormalities stem from genetic inheritance or age, but in most cases their cause is unknown. Environmental factors such as long-term exposure to pesticides,[21] cigarette smoking, exposure to job-related toxins (heavy metals and industrial chemicals), and excessive heat or cold are likely to play roles. So, too, are free radical damage and oxidative stress.[2]

More research is necessary to conclusively determine the causes of sperm cell abnormalities and male infertility. But according to what we know about oxidative damage, sperm cells probably are very susceptible to DNA alterations by free radicals, leading to faulty replication. This may be why Mother Nature has equipped men with accessory sex glands that secrete antioxidant enzymes into seminal fluid: The secretions may help to protect sperm against oxidative damage.[9] Recent animal research shows that taking antioxidant supplements—including vitamin C, vitamin E, and isoflavones—may have a similar protective effect.[8, 24]

As we've thought about the tradition of presenting bouquets of *Rhodiola rosea* root to Georgian and Siberian brides, we've realized that when a woman brews tea from the root, she likely serves it to her husband in addition to drinking a cup herself. So the herb may enhance fertility in both partners—in the man, by increasing stress resistance and reducing oxidative damage to sperm DNA.

A good next step would be to test *Rhodiola rosea* and other powerful adaptogens that have shown positive effects on fertility and semen quality to see whether they could improve sperm quality as well. If so, the list of *Rhodiola rosea*'s benefits might grow to include improved male and female fertility, fewer miscarriages, and—possibly—the prevention of certain birth defects and childhood cancers.

THE BIG PICTURE

Many of our patients, as well as those of our colleagues, have reported that they are enjoying a more satisfying sex life and deeper intimacy with their partners, thanks to *Rhodiola rosea*. Of course, no single treatment works for everyone. Often in our own practices, we combine the best of both worlds—prescription medications and healing herbs—to get optimal results. You, too, should think twice before putting all of your eggs, or sperm, in one basket.

Remember, healthy sexual function depends on many variables. By the same token, sexual *dys*function can have any number of causes—including too much stress, not enough sleep, unresolved emotional problems, interpersonal conflicts, or unhealthy habits such as smoking cigarettes. So before you rush out to buy *Rhodiola rosea*, Viagra, or anything else to enhance your sexual desire and response, take stock of all the factors that may be contributing to your situation and address those that won't be cured with a pill.

How to take Rhodiola rosea . . .

TO IMPROVE SEXUAL DESIRE AND RESPONSE

Start by taking one 100-milligram capsule of Rhodiola rosea *½ hour before breakfast on an empty stomach. As long as you don't feel overstimulated or have difficulty sleeping, you can add another capsule every 3 to 7 days until you see results. If you reach a total of four capsules daily—two before breakfast and two before lunch—stay at that dosage for at least a month to see the full effects. If after 1 month you don't notice any difference, take a third capsule before breakfast. Wait at least 2 more weeks, and if necessary, add a third capsule before lunch. This is your maximum dosage: six capsules per day.*

If you feel "revved up" and you're also consuming caffeine, then cut back on coffee, black tea, and caffeinated soft drinks. If overstimulation continues to be a problem, you may need to temporarily reduce your dosage of Rhodiola rosea *so you can build your tolerance more gradually. You can do this by adding one-half of a capsule to your dose every 2 weeks.*

CHAPTER 12

Restore
HORMONAL
BALANCE

Like the weather, the female body is subject to constant change. The internal storms—as well as periods of calm—are driven by fluctuations in estrogen and progesterone, both female sex hormones. The amounts of these hormones produced by the ovaries rise and fall, not just according to the different phases of the menstrual cycle but also in relation to a woman's stage of life. For example, the onset of menstruation ushers in its own particular set of hormonal changes, as do premenopause and menopause—all superimposed on the ups and downs of the monthly cycle.

Of course, no two women are exactly alike, even in their degree of sensitivity to hormonal fluctuations. Some may experience severe mood swings or fatigue, while others complain primarily of bloating and cramps. Still others may feel only intermittent discomforts. But no matter what their individual experiences, most women must figure out how to manage hormonal changes at some point in their lives, whether they're grappling with premenstrual syndrome—the infamous PMS—or the erratic menstrual cycles typical of perimenopause.

RHODIOLA ROSEA:
NATURE'S HORMONE HELPER

Many women find that *Rhodiola rosea* helps to offset certain hormone-related symptoms. For instance, the herb can reduce the fatigue, irritability, and depression that occur during the premenstrual and menstrual phases. For a woman in perimenopause, *Rhodiola rosea* is effective at improving energy, mental clarity, memory, and mood. It also seems to normalize menstrual cycles and certain physical changes, such as vaginal dryness, although we're not exactly sure how it does this.

PMS AND PMDD

While not all women have heard of PMDD, which stands for premenstrual dysphoric disorder, most are familiar with PMS. This is because sooner or later most women experience some of the physiological and behavioral changes associated with the female menstrual cycle. Estimates of the number of women who struggle with PMS vary wildly, with some experts putting the figure as high as 90 percent. The American College of Obstetricians and Gynecologists estimates that 20 to 40 percent of women experience significant premenstrual discomforts, with another 5 percent suffering from PMDD, a depressive illness.

Suzanne had struggled with severe PMS for most of her life. In general, she was a happy, enthusiastic person—except the week before her periods, when her hormone levels dropped. That's when she seemed to undergo the sort of dramatic personality change made famous by Dr. Jekyll and his evil counterpart, Mr. Hyde. During that 1 week every month, she became short-tempered, critical, anxious, and moody, to the point where she claimed to feel like a victim of demonic possession.

Pat was able to rein in Suzanne's PMS with antidepressants. But as Suzanne approached menopause, her symptoms came back with a vengeance. Once again, she found herself screaming at her husband and children. After trying every possible standard treatment, Pat prescribed 500 milligrams daily of *Rhodiola rosea*. Sure enough, it banished Suzanne's hormonal demons.

WHEN MENSTRUAL CYCLES GO MISSING

A woman's menstrual cycle can stop for many reasons other than pregnancy or menopause. For example, malnutrition, anorexia, stress, illness, and hormone imbalance are known to contribute to the cessation of monthly periods. The term *primary amenorrhea* applies to women who never began menstruating in the first place—usually because of an anatomical, hormonal, or genetic disorder, or severe malnutrition. *Secondary amenorrhea* refers to women who miss three or more periods after having had regular menstrual cycles.

In a Soviet study involving 40 women—seven with primary amenorrhea, 33 with secondary amenorrhea—scientists administered *Rhodiola rosea* either by mouth or by injection for 10 to 14 days. In some cases, they repeated the treatment several times. The herb successfully restored normal periods in 25 of the women. Of these, 11 subsequently became pregnant.[4, 7]

While this particular study is intriguing, it lacks sufficient scientific detail for us to fully interpret the results. Nevertheless, in our own clinical experience, treatment with *Rhodiola rosea* appears just as promising. We've seen the herb successfully restore regular monthly menstrual cycles in several of our premenopausal and menopausal patients who had missed their periods for more than 6 months.

Two of Dick's patients, women in their early forties, had failed to become pregnant after 2 years of in vitro fertilization and synthetic hormones. Within 3 months of stopping all hormonal treatments and starting *Rhodiola rosea*, 300 milligrams a day, both women not only became pregnant but also carried to term and bore healthy babies. The possibility that *Rhodiola rosea* might increase the chances of pregnancy in women with fertility problems is worthy of further research.

THE PERIMENOPAUSE CHALLENGE

Many women entering perimenopause—with the initial onset usually around age 40—seek our help for the anxiety, depression, memory problems, and sexual disorders that tend to go with the territory. We have found that in terms of treatment, one size does not fit all. So we do our best to tailor our recommendations to each patient. Understanding the particular physical changes and psychological issues that a woman faces is essential to developing an effective treatment plan.

Sometimes our bottom-line prescription simply is more rest. Women need to recognize that after age 40, they require more downtime to rejuvenate their bodies. For some, especially those whose careers might just be taking off, this can be a bitter pill to swallow. Poor diet, lack of exercise, and other bad habits, such as smoking and excessive alcohol consumption—which may not have caused problems in the past—start showing their effects as well. There isn't any way around it: As a woman gets older, her body needs ample doses of rest, nutritional supplements (including vitamins and antioxidants), and physical activity in order to stay healthy.

Though we may not think twice about it when we're young, maintaining our cellular energy reserves becomes a major challenge as we get older. Our cellular repair mechanisms simply can't protect us from oxidative damage as well as they once did. The liver can't detoxify substances such as alcohol as easily, and as a result, brain cells succumb more readily to the toxic effects of alcohol and recreational drugs.

The added strain of illness and the effects of medications—part and parcel of the aging process—must be taken into account. So, too, must our overall life situations, including the quality of our relationships and the burden of our responsibilities. All of these factors influence emotional and physical health—and, in women, the experience of perimenopause and menopause.

Most women in perimenopause or beyond benefit from a combination of approaches that may include dietary changes, nutritional supplementation, exercise, relaxation training, psychotherapy, medication, and—when appropriate—*Rhodiola rosea*. We've found that many of our female patients age 40 and older respond positively to the herb, experiencing greater energy, sharper mental function and memory, and better mood.

MAKING PEACE WITH "THE CHANGE"

For Betty, menopause came on with hot flashes, drenching night sweats, insomnia, weight gain, anxiety, and low-grade depression. In other words, she got the worst of it. Fortunately, Dick was able to relieve all of her symptoms with a winning combination: Bio-Strath, a rich blend of B vitamins and antioxidants; Remifemin, made from an herb called black cohosh; and 400 milligrams daily of *Rhodiola rosea*.

With this treatment regimen, Betty's hot flashes and night sweats stopped almost immediately. Her depression and anxiety lifted over the next several months. She slept well, and when she woke up in the morning, she looked forward to the day ahead. To her great relief, once her symptoms subsided, she had no trouble losing the extra pounds she had gained.

While some women look forward to menopause as a respite from a lifetime of menstrual cycles, most await it with a combination of wariness and dread. It raises the specter of a whole host of challenges to the body, mind, and spirit: diminishing health, including an increased risk of heart disease, cancer, and osteoporosis; lack of sexual desire and response; decline in memory and mental ability; erosion or loss of personal relationships. These challenges seem even more daunting now that the dream of synthetic hormone replacement therapy (HRT) as a way to stay young and feminine has turned into a nightmare.

Long-term studies that identified HRT as a risk factor for breast and uterine cancers have left most women wondering what they can do to preserve their health and vitality for as long as possible.[1, 6] Few want to gamble on HRT, even in lower doses—especially since claims of protective effects against heart disease and dementia have turned out to be untrue.[5] In fact, the very latest research suggests that HRT actually *raises* the risk of heart disease and dementia.[8, 9] But if not HRT to manage menopause, then what?

A growing number of women are turning to natural remedies—such as the plant estrogens in soy, black cohosh (*Cimicifuga racemosa*), and chasteberry or vitex (*Vitex agnus-castus*)—to ease the menopausal transition. Because they're natural, plant estrogens (also called phytoestrogens) are believed to be safer and milder than synthetic hormone replacement. But this has yet to be confirmed by long-term large-scale studies.

In the United Sates, pharmaceutical companies support most medication research and development. Because they really can't earn a profit from natural substances, which they can't patent, they're reluctant to fund studies on plant estrogens. Fortunately, many medical centers are helping to bridge this research gap by establishing departments of complementary and alternative medicine. At the Rosenthal Center of Columbia University, for example, scientists are conducting studies of black cohosh and other phytoestrogens.

CONFIRMING THE SAFETY
OF *RHODIOLA ROSEA*

Pat: We are aware of populations—mainly villagers in the mountains of Siberia and the Republic of Georgia—who take *Rhodiola rosea* every day throughout their lives without any increase in their risk of cancer. This epidemiological information has reassured us about the safety of the herb. What's more, numerous studies have suggested that *Rhodiola rosea* actually has anticarcinogenic properties, which we'll discuss further in chapter 13.

Rhodiola rosea in the Research Spotlight

Patricia Eagon, M.D., Ph.D., a professor at the University of Pittsburgh Medical Center, and her laboratory assistants, Frank Houghton, Ph.D., and Mary Elm, investigated whether *Rhodiola rosea* would stimulate uterine growth—an indicator of estrogenic action and also of potential uterine cancer risk. To do so, they used a standard laboratory procedure to surgically induce menopause in a group of female rats. Just as with menopausal women, the rats' uteruses shrank with the sudden drop in circulating estrogen. Then Dr. Eagon and her colleagues fed the rats 65 milligrams of *Rhodiola rosea* daily, one-fourth the usual therapeutic dose for women. The herb did not stimulate uterine growth—a very good sign of safety, especially since 65 milligrams is a large dose for such small animals.

Another aspect of the study involved assessing sensitivity to estrogenic substances. Normally the pituitary gland produces luteinizing hormone (LH) to stimulate the ovaries to release estrogen, which in turn stimulates the uterus to enlarge in preparation for possible pregnancy. If an ovum (egg) goes unfertilized, estrogen feeds back to the pituitary, telling it to reduce production of LH. In fact, during menopause both women and rats have high levels of circulating LH because of the decline in estrogen.

In Dr. Eagon's study, *Rhodiola rosea* did not act on the pituitary or cause a drop in LH, nor did it elevate estradiol E2—all excellent signs that *Rhodiola rosea* would not stimulate uterine growth. Even the very sensitive endocrine systems of the rats—which received a dose of the herb many times larger than humans normally would, in proportion to their size—did not react to

---

Nevertheless, the lack of hard scientific data concerned me. How could I recommend *Rhodiola rosea* to my menopausal patients without knowing more definitively how it might affect them in 10 or 20 years? All I could say to them was that the risk of cancer probably is low, but the herb hasn't been thoroughly tested. What's more, even though I had seen several breast cancer survivors do quite well with *Rhodiola rosea*, I didn't feel comfortable using the herb to treat women with a history of estrogen-sensitive cancers.

When I learned that it's possible to evaluate compounds for cancer risk by testing their estrogenic effects on uterine growth, breast tissue,

---

Rhodiola rosea as an estrogenic substance. In other words, *Rhodiola rosea* is unlikely to increase uterine cancer risk.

Dr. Eagon and her colleagues also evaluated the potential effects of *Rhodiola rosea* on breast cells. The first round of tests found that in the large doses fed to rats, the herb has strong estrogen receptor–binding properties. But these tests did not distinguish between molecules that activate the receptors (estrogens) and those that inactivate the receptors (anti-estrogens, such as tamoxifen). They simply showed an interaction.

In the second round of tests, Dr. Eagon and her research team outfitted menopausal rats with estradiol (E2) implants, similar to the Norplant contraceptive. The implants released an above-normal amount of the hormone into the animals' bloodstream. The rats that were fed *Rhodiola rosea* showed 10 to 20 percent lower levels of circulating estradiol than the rats that were not fed the herb. *Rhodiola rosea* brought abnormally high levels of the hormone toward normal.

The results imply that women using estrogen replacement or oral contraceptives need not worry that *Rhodiola rosea* will elevate estradiol because the herb appears to reduce the hormone when levels climb too high. By the same token, menopausal or postmenopausal women and breast cancer patients can feel more comfortable taking *Rhodiola rosea* because in therapeutic doses it does not produce an estrogenic effect.[2, 3]

and breast cancer cells, I contacted Patricia Eagon, M.D., Ph.D., a professor at the University of Pittsburgh Medical Center who's an expert on estrogen receptor testing. Dr. Eagon was about to launch another round of extensive testing, and she agreed to add *Rhodiola rosea* to her experiments. (I will summarize her key findings here. For a more detailed discussion of her research protocol, see page 180.)

A compound with an estrogenic effect can increase uterine cancer risk if it stimulates uterine growth. In laboratory studies involving menopausal rats, Dr. Eagon discovered that *Rhodiola rosea* does not stimulate uterine growth, even in very large doses. Nor does the herb have an estrogenic effect on the pituitary gland.

Dr. Eagon also determined that *Rhodiola rosea* does not decrease the level of luteinizing hormone (LH). Produced by the pituitary gland, LH stimulates the ovaries to release estradiol, a form of estrogen. Estradiol then circulates in the bloodstream, alerting the pituitary when to slow production of LH. A compound with an estrogenic effect will do the same thing, causing a drop in the amount of LH that is circulating in the bloodstream. So by measuring the LH level in blood samples, scientists can measure the estrogenic effect of a particular compound.

When uterine and breast tissues are subjected to excess estrogen for many years, as is the case with hormone replacement therapy, they are more likely to become cancerous. For the same reason, a compound with an estrogenic effect can increase uterine and breast cancer risk over time. Given the outcome of Dr. Eagon's experiments, which found no increase in uterine growth and no drop in LH levels (meaning no estrogenic effect), *Rhodiola rosea* seems unlikely to increase uterine cancer risk.

With this encouraging finding, Dr. Eagon and I were eager to find out whether *Rhodiola rosea* would stimulate or suppress breast cell growth. Dr. Eagon's testing showed that the herb does bind to estrogen receptors. But in rats fitted with estradiol implants (which elevate the hormone above normal), *Rhodiola rosea* lowered blood estradiol levels by 10 to 20 percent. This suggests an absence of estrogenic effect—another indicator of the herb's safety for menopausal women and possibly breast cancer patients.

Currently, Dr. Eagon's team is evaluating how *Rhodiola rosea* influences breast cancer cells growing in cultures. We hope to hear more about this exciting research in the years ahead. [2, 3]

࿇

How to take Rhodiola rosea . . .

TO BALANCE HORMONES

Try taking 100 milligrams of Rhodiola rosea *½ hour before breakfast on an empty stomach for several days to see how it affects your system. If you feel overstimulated, you may need to reduce your dosage—say, to one-quarter or one-half of a capsule—and increase your tolerance more gradually. On the other hand, if you experience no problems after 5 days, take a second capsule ½ hour before lunch. Wait about a week to see how you feel. If you think you need more, then add another capsule before breakfast.*

After a month or so, you should be able to assess how well this regimen is working and whether you would benefit from taking a second capsule before lunch. Most women need 300 to 400 milligrams a day of Rhodiola rosea *to balance their hormones, though some need as much as 600 milligrams. Allow at least a month after each increase above 400 milligrams to see results.*

Jump-Start Your
DISEASE
DEFENSES

Cancer is a pressing national priority. So many lives have been touched by the disease, directly and indirectly, that nonprofit organizations across the country raise millions of dollars every year for cancer research. Despite the many lifesaving treatments that have emerged, however, the national cancer rate continues to climb. And while the economic cost of surgery, chemotherapy, and radiation is high, the human cost in suffering from side effects and illnesses secondary to treatment is beyond measure.

Cancer begins with changes in chromosomal DNA. Changes to chromosomes occur all the time. Most are benign, meaning that they don't lead to cancer. But some can cause normal cells to mutate into cancer cells.

Anything that can cause normal cells to become cancerous is referred to as *mutagenic* or *carcinogenic*. Common carcinogens include radiation, excessive sun exposure, environmental toxins (such as pesticides, asbestos, and industrial waste), cigarette smoke, chemicals, medications, hepatitis and other infections, charred or "blackened" foods, and trans fatty acids. Genetic vulnerability also plays a role in individual cancer risk.

We can substantially reduce our cancer risk by avoiding exposure to some carcinogens—such as cigarette smoke and the sun's ultraviolet rays—and minimizing exposure to others. For example, we can eat organic foods to avoid hazardous pesticides, chemicals, and hormones. On a larger scale, we can support efforts to clean up industrial waste sites and to keep our air, water, and soil as pure as possible. Measures like these will provide long-term protection from carcinogens for us as well as for future generations.

ANTIOXIDANTS: THE FRONT LINE IN THE FIGHT AGAINST CANCER

Another smart strategy in the fight against cancer is to increase our intake of nutrients with proven anticarcinogenic and antioxidant properties. Lately, as you no doubt have noticed, antioxidant supplements have become all the rage. Part of the reason is that antioxidants prevent the free radical damage to cellular DNA that sets the stage for cancer-causing cellular mutations.

Carcinogens harm DNA and other cellular components through a variety of mechanisms. Cigarette smoke, for example, contains free radicals that spread through the lungs every time the smoker inhales. Free radicals from tobacco also dissolve in saliva, which puts them in contact with the mouth, throat, esophagus, and (after swallowing) stomach. The energy from carcinogens such as x-rays or ultraviolet radiation strikes molecules in the skin, creating free radicals that split off and cause skin cancer—including melanoma, the most dangerous kind—as well as age spots, wrinkles, and general skin aging. Other carcinogens, such as pesticides, cause free radical damage when the body tries to metabolize and detoxify them.

Antioxidants neutralize free radicals before they attack cellular DNA. Nature's primary source of antioxidants is plant-derived foods, especially fruits and vegetables. Why do plants contain antioxidants? Because like any living thing, they need to protect and repair themselves.

For example, plants absorb their energy from the sun—and in the process, they sustain free radical damage from the sun's ultraviolet rays. Over time, they've evolved mechanisms to produce a myriad of antioxidant compounds. Some plants that grow at very high altitudes, like *Rhodiola rosea*, contain the most powerful antioxidants—possibly because they must survive in the most challenging environments, with high-intensity sunlight, extreme cold, harsh winds, low oxygen, and a brief growing season.

Learning which fruits and vegetables contain an abundance of antioxidants and eating a variety of them every day provides broad-spectrum protection against many of the carcinogens in our environment. We can further boost our antioxidant defenses by taking supplements made from plants, such as *Rhodiola rosea*, that you won't find in the produce aisle.

Antioxidant supplements are widely available in supermarkets, drugstores, and health food stores, as well as on the Internet. So how do you choose from among so many brands? What makes one product better than the rest?

There are two things you need to know when choosing an antioxidant supplement. First, many products currently on the market are poorly absorbed in the stomach. This means that most of what you swallow never actually gets into your system. Second, many products have not undergone adequate testing to determine whether they contain antioxidants in the amounts stated on the label and whether they actually do what they claim. So before you buy an antioxidant supplement, try to find out whether any scientific studies have confirmed its effectiveness.

On page 229, you will find product recommendations for all the supplements that we mention in this book. Additional sources of unbiased information include the American Botanical Council, the Natural Medicines Comprehensive Database, and consumerlab.com. For further information on these resources, see page 227.

We prescribe *Rhodiola rosea* because research has shown that it contains compounds with strong antioxidant properties and is well absorbed in the stomach.[3, 7] We've listed sources of good-quality *Rhodiola rosea* products on page 230. All of these products have been tested and standardized to contain at least 3.0 percent rosavins and at least 1.0 percent salidroside.

DUAL BENEFITS FOR DNA

Rhodiola rosea not only reduces cellular free radical damage, it also appears to improve DNA repair, another factor in preventing cancer. Breaks in DNA strands are actually quite common and usually harmless. But trouble can occur during the repair process, when errors (mutations) in the patched-up DNA can replicate and generate more cancer cells.

After a DNA strand splits, the gap between the two sides widens, just like a tear in your favorite sweater. Ideally, the gap will knit back together without disruption in the DNA pattern. Participating in this repair process are two competing enzymes: polymerase and exonuclease. Polymerase reduces the size of the gap, and the chances of defective repair, better than exonuclease. So when polymerase dominates the repair process, carcinogenic defects are less likely to occur. *Rhodiola rosea* promotes the activity of polymerase, which may improve the quality of DNA repair and minimize the frequency of mutations.[12]

In studies of mice injected with a carcinogen called cyclophosphamide, *Rhodiola rosea* reduced the development of chromosomal and cellular aberrations by 50 percent. And in mice given N-nitroso-N-methylurea, a carcinogen that damages DNA and causes bone marrow cells to turn cancerous, *Rhodiola rosea* promoted DNA repair and prevented cell mutation.[12]

Many other animal studies show that the herb has antimutagenic, anticarcinogenic, and antimetastatic benefits. (*Antimetastatic* means that it stops cancer from spreading.) *Rhodiola rosea* also appears to protect normal cells from radiation damage, as well as from chemotherapy toxicity.[10]

ENHANCING THE EFFECTIVENESS OF CHEMOTHERAPY

Like a military shock-and-awe campaign, most cancer treatments aim to destroy cancer cells while minimizing damage to healthy cells, in the hope that the "civilian" cellular population will survive and recover from the devastation. But even as researchers rush to find new treatments that will selectively destroy cancer cells while sparing healthy tissues, patients continue to suffer collateral damage.

Two of the most hazardous side effects of cancer treatment are liver toxicity and bone marrow suppression. Chemotherapy damage to bone marrow stem cells can cause bleeding, anemia, and loss of immune defenses.

After Yumiko, a 58-year-old martial arts instructor, underwent a mastectomy for breast cancer, chemotherapy caused such severe drops in her white and red blood cell counts that her doctor repeatedly suspended her treatment. Like many cancer patients, she felt caught in a deadly bind in which the therapy can be as bad as the disease.

Yumiko consulted Dick, who recommended taking 150 milligrams of *Rhodiola rosea* twice a day. The herb normalized her white and red blood counts and kept them within an acceptable range during a complete—and successful—course of chemotherapy. What's more, *Rhodiola rosea* gave Yumiko the energy she needed to return to teaching the martial arts, which she loves.

Mel always had been a healthy man, very independent and upbeat, until he developed chronic lymphocytic leukemia—an abnormal proliferation of white blood cells—in his seventies. Standard chemotherapy proved disastrous. The drugs suppressed Mel's bone marrow stem cells and caused a precipitous drop in his white cells, red cells, and platelets, which are essential for blood clotting. The destruction of Mel's immune defenses led to septic shock, a critical and potentially life-threatening infection that invades the bloodstream.

When the oncologist informed Mel's family that his condition was terminal and he had no more than 2 months to live, his daughter got in touch with Dick, who prescribed two adaptogens: *Rhodiola rosea* and *Eleutheroccus senticosus*. Mel's strength, energy, and outlook improved almost immediately, and the sepsis cleared up in 3 weeks. The addition of shark liver oil and cat's claw (*Uncaria tomentosa*)—another herb that supports DNA repair—stabilized Mel's leukemia, reducing the number of abnormal white blood cells while raising the number of red cells and platelets.

One year later, thinking he was cured, Mel stopped taking the herbs without telling Dick. Soon he developed a septic staph infection that remained unresponsive to antibiotics for 4 weeks. The medication kicked in only after he went back on the adaptogens and began taking other immune boosters—astragalus and a mixture of 12 medicinal mushrooms.

The herbal regimen worked; eventually, Mel was free from all infection. He surprised his family by living another year—nearly 2 years beyond the original 2-month prognosis.

Rhodiola rosea appears to reduce toxic damage to the liver and to bone marrow, our renewable source of blood cells.[14, 15, 16] In animal studies, the combination of *Rhodiola rosea* and chemotherapy drugs destroys more cancer cells and does a better job of preventing metastases than either treatment alone. The beauty of the herb is that it increases the effectiveness of anticancer drugs while reducing their toxicity to healthy cells.

RELIEF AND RECOVERY

Besides improving chemotherapy and protecting the liver and bone marrow, *Rhodiola rosea* can alleviate other symptoms that often plague cancer patients. These include fatigue, anxiety, depression, and stress, with fatigue being the most frequent and distressing complaint. In fact, fatigue can linger for months or even years after the cancer has gone because the treatment is so intense.[17]

Eleanor, a public relations consultant, was diagnosed with breast cancer at age 53. Following a lumpectomy, she underwent radiation and chemotherapy. The treatments left her so exhausted that she could barely walk. She took a leave of absence from work and spent most of her time just sitting around the house. Even though her appetite was almost nonexistent, her inactivity resulted in a weight gain of 50 pounds.

Dick, whom Eleanor had previously consulted for depression,

prescribed 200 milligrams of *Rhodiola rosea* twice a day. Gradually, over a 2-month period, her energy returned. She felt well enough to undertake an exercise program and quickly lost 30 pounds. Not long after, she eagerly returned to work.

Depression, another common complaint among cancer patients, frequently goes hand in hand with fatigue.

Renee—a psychologist whom Dick had successfully treated for depression and fibromyalgia—was doing well until shortly after her 48th birthday, when a mammogram detected breast cancer that had infiltrated her chest wall. After a mastectomy, radiation, and chemotherapy, Renee felt overwhelmed with fatigue. What's more, her depression came back full force. A daily dose of 400 milligrams of *Rhodiola rosea* dramatically improved both her energy and her mood.

All went well for a year, until a follow-up mammogram revealed cancer in Renee's remaining breast. Naturally, she became upset and depressed. She couldn't imagine going through another mastectomy. Dick doubled her dose of *Rhodiola rosea*, which sustained her mood and energy through the second surgery and course of chemotherapy. She continues to take the herb and now is fully engaged in her work and personal life.

Unfortunately, very few oncologists—or medical doctors in general—know about *Rhodiola rosea*. When patients suggest it, most physicians won't allow it, for fear that it will somehow compromise the action of chemotherapy drugs. While this can happen with certain herbs as well as with certain medications, it is not the case with *Rhodiola rosea*, according to the numerous studies that we've cited here.

Nevertheless, though the existing research is promising, more is needed to determine the full potential of *Rhodiola rosea* as an adjunct to chemotherapy. Perhaps such studies would help persuade physicians that the herb is safe for cancer patients.

COMPELLING EVIDENCE
FROM THE LAB

Some of the most notorious bacteria around are put to work in the laboratory by scientists testing potential cancer treatments. In one study, for example, *Rhodiola rosea* protected salmonella strains from a dozen different carcinogens. In some cases, the protective effect was as high as 90 percent.[5] Another study used *Escherichia coli* bacteria to screen substances with the potential to keep cells from mutating. Once again, *Rhodiola rosea* passed with flying colors, demonstrating high general protective effects and specific antimutagenic activity.[6]

Often scientists test cancer treatments by transplanting human cancer cells into mice, then administering various chemotherapy drugs. In four kinds of transplanted tumors, including melanoma, *Rhodiola rosea* showed both antitumor and antimetastatic properties. And when the mice received chemotherapy, *Rhodiola rosea* increased their survival rate.[4]

Cyclophosphamide is the double-edged sword of cancer treatment: A powerful cancer drug, it also causes DNA damage in bone marrow stem cells. When researchers injected two groups of mice with different types of cancer cells, treatment with cyclophosphamide suppressed tumor growth by 31 to 39 percent and metastases by 18 percent. Unfortunately, it significantly reduced the number of normal white blood cells in bone marrow as well.

Then the researchers tried *Rhodiola rosea*. Like cyclophosphamide, the herb significantly suppressed tumor growth and metastases, though not as much as the drug. On the other hand, it didn't deplete healthy bone marrow stem cells, either. So the researchers combined *Rhodiola rosea* and cyclophosphamide, with even better results. The combination not only boosted antimetastatic activity by 36 percent, it also increased the number of bone marrow stem cells and leukocytes, a type of white blood cell.[14]

At this time, we're aware of only one published study of *Rhodiola rosea* in cancer patients. In the study, which involved 12 people with superficial bladder cancer, the herb improved leukocyte and T cell immunity. Although the patients who took *Rhodiola rosea* were less likely to experience a relapse, the difference did not reach statistical significance, perhaps because the study was so small.[1] Meanwhile, researchers in Moscow are planning a clinical trial to examine *Rhodiola rosea*'s ability to prevent chemotherapy side effects.

IMMUNE SYSTEM SUPPORT

The immune system offers another line of defense against cancer. Sometimes as cells begin to mutate and become cancerous, the immune system identifies them as abnormal and destroys them before they develop into a more robust form of the disease. This is one reason that a compromised immune system can increase the body's susceptibility to cancer. Reinforcing your immune defenses provides extra protection against cancer, not to mention a host of other illnesses.

Long before research established that *Rhodiola rosea* enhances immune defense mechanisms within cells, people in the mountain villages of eastern Russia and Siberia—as well as in central Asia and Scandinavia—relied on the herb to help fight infections. During the harsh Siberian winters, villagers brewed *Rhodiola rosea* tea to treat colds and flu, while Mongolian doctors prescribed it for tuberculosis and cancer. In Norway, doctors routinely used the herb as a treatment for scurvy, lung disease, and intestinal worms.[9]

As animal studies show, *Rhodiola rosea* can stimulate the natural killer cells that protect against infections. Natural killer cells originate in the thymus gland and migrate to the lymph nodes, liver, spleen, and gastrointestinal tract—pretty much all over the body. A large pool of them exist in a rat's liver, while the human liver has a proportionately smaller number. In one study, removing part of the rats' livers caused a decline in natural killer cells. Yet after the rats received five injections of *Rhodiola rosea*, natural killer cell activity in the gastrointestinal tract rose by 112 percent. With 12 injections, cell activity in the spleen shot up by 222 percent.[2]

In 1998, Andrey Yaremenko—then an enterprising graduate student at the I. P. Pavlov St. Petersburg State Medical University in Russia—presented "The Complex Treatment of Severe Infectious Diseases," his Ph.D. dissertation in medicine. Through his research, he had determined that *Rhodiola rosea* could destroy pathogenic bacteria in cell cultures as effectively as the antibiotic oxacillin. In rats with staphylococcus infections of the jaw, the herb worked as well as another antibiotic, bicillin. In fact, it reduced ESR (erythrocyte sedimentation rate)—an indicator of inflammation—better than the drug.

The combination of bicillin and *Rhodiola rosea* appeared to be even more effective. In a controlled study involving 200 patients hospitalized with acute, severe infections that had begun in a tooth and spread to the mouth, face, and neck, half of the patients received standard treatment, while the rest also received a concentrated alcohol extract of *Rhodiola rosea*. After doctors drained the infected teeth, patients with a favorable prognosis did well while using *Rhodiola rosea* alone. Those with more questionable prognoses took a course of antibiotics. The patients who combined their antibiotics with *Rhodiola rosea* recovered faster than those who didn't.

In the most severe cases, those with unfavorable prognoses, treatment consisted of surgical drainage, antibiotics, diuresis to prevent toxic shock, and low-intensity laser irradiation of the blood. Even for these severely ill patients, *Rhodiola rosea* accelerated recovery by rapidly reducing inflammation, enhancing detoxification, and normalizing the cellular immune response.[18]

STRESS, DEPRESSION, AND DISEASE

Rhodiola rosea also may support the immune system by protecting against the adverse effects of stress and depression, which can impair immune function and increase vulnerability to infections and cancer. Research has shown that stressful events—bereavement, divorce, and academic exams—suppress immunity.[11] When we're stressed-out, we are more likely to fall victim to one of the many cold or flu viruses

---

What Every Parent Should Know

When students get stressed during final exams, their levels of natural killer cells and lymphocytes decline, which increases their chances of contracting illnesses such as mononucleosis or activating latent viruses such as herpes. Fortunately, most of them can survive a few weeks of intense studying and testing without getting sick. Their immune defenses return to normal once the exam period is over.[8, 11]

Some students, though, are more vulnerable to infections. What's more, research has linked chronic academic stress with susceptibility to "mono," which can lead to months of fatigue and diminished academic performance.

Help is available in the form of *Rhodiola rosea*, which can reduce stress and fatigue during exam periods.[13] If you have a student in college who tends to get run-down or stressed-out, you might consider tucking a bottle of the herb into the care package that you send around exam time. Be sure to include clear instructions to start with one 100-milligram capsule and to wait 3 to 7 days before adding another.

Most students do not need more than one or two capsules a day; they should not exceed four a day. If they drink a lot of caffeine, they should cut back while taking *Rhodiola rosea* to avoid feeling jittery.

---

that seem to be everywhere around us. A cough, a sore throat, a stuffy nose—these are the body's way of saying that its resistance is low.

While short-term, acute stress actually can bolster the immune system, chronic stress has the opposite effect, hampering immune function over time. This is because stress activates the HPA (hypothalamic-pituitary-adrenal) axis, which in turn increases the production of adrenal glucocorticoids. It also stimulates the sympathetic nervous system, causing a rise in epinephrine and norepinephrine. Excessive or sustained release of all these hormones can suppress immunity. Fortunately, *Rhodiola rosea* helps to counteract their effects.

How to take Rhodiola rosea . . .

AS AN IMMUNE BOOSTER
Start by taking one 100-milligram capsule of Rhodiola rosea *in the morning, ½ hour before breakfast, on an empty stomach. If after 3 days you're able to tolerate this dose, add a second capsule ½ hour before lunch. Most people don't need more than 200 milligrams per day unless they're sick or fatigued. If necessary, you can increase your dosage after another 3 to 7 days with a second capsule before breakfast and, after another week, with a second capsule before lunch—for a total of 400 milligrams daily. You can stay at this dosage as long as you don't feel overstimulated.*

CHAPTER 14

Drop
EXCESS
POUNDS

Health care professionals have declared a national state of emergency. The reason: Nearly two-thirds of American adults are overweight, with half of this population qualifying as obese. When you consider all of the health implications of these statistics—most notably a significant increase in the death rate from all causes—the magnitude of our nation's weight problem becomes clear.

Admittedly, you needn't be right at your ideal weight in order to be healthy. But the closer you are to that number, the less likely you are to develop an obesity-related illness such as heart disease, high blood pressure, diabetes, or cancer. If you're more than 30 percent—roughly 30 to 50 pounds—above your ideal weight, it's in your best interest to take steps to turn around your situation. This is especially true if you have a family history of heart disease or diabetes, or if you already are showing signs of cardiovascular disease or high blood pressure. On the other hand, if you're more than 10 percent *below* your ideal weight, that can be a health hazard, too.

WHY WE GAIN

There are many factors that contribute to weight gain. And there are just as many diets and exercise programs that promise to melt away the extra pounds. We are not offering a quick fix or embracing a fad—whether it's high-protein low-carb, low-protein high-carb, grapefruit-only, or something else. For in the battle of the bulge, it's our responsibility as health care professionals to acknowledge the challenges of staying trim.

For most of us, the pounds creep up slowly as we alternate between resisting and succumbing to our weaknesses and cravings. We may eat mindfully all day, carefully counting every calorie and avoiding sweets. Then, late at night when we're feeling stressed or exhausted, we reach for the potato chips or the pint of Ben & Jerry's. Just like that, our good intentions go out the window. "Tomorrow," we promise ourselves as we devour our favorite treats. "Tomorrow I'll be good."

Seeking comfort in food is human nature—which, unfortunately, makes losing weight all the more challenging. Our first step must be to stop blaming ourselves. Self-blame is counterproductive. The worse you feel about yourself, the more you want to eat to escape. Caring about yourself and your health, and about the welfare of those you love, is a far better way to motivate yourself to make changes.

What's more, many of us are conditioned to eat as though we still live in a nation of farmers who spend 10 hours a day tilling the land. We need to adapt our dietary habits to conform to our modern, more sedentary lifestyle. We can't eat like our parents or grandparents, many of whom were physically active from the time the sun rose in the morning until it set in the evening.

Get with the Program

Some people have the self-discipline to take off 5 or 10 pounds by dieting and exercising. But the majority—particularly those who are more than 30 percent above their ideal weight—need a structured weight-loss plan. Fortunately, this kind of help is everywhere. You can ask your doctor or another health care professional to help create a plan just for you. Or join an organization such as Weight Watchers or Overeaters Anonymous. Many hospitals sponsor weight-loss clinics as well.

If you're too busy or too uncomfortable to attend meetings in person, there are weight-loss programs that allow you to check in by phone. One is operated by Health Management Resources. To learn more, call 800-418-1367 or visit the company's Web site at www.hmrathome.com. Another good Web site is www.ornish.com, the Internet home of world-renowned cardiologist Dean Ornish, M.D. The site offers scientifically sound dietary advice, as well as research updates that are particularly relevant for heart health.

In chapter 15, we'll present our guidelines for a healthy, high-energy diet that will help move you toward your ideal weight. Here we will focus our attention on the relationship between stress, low energy, and weight gain—and the potentially pivotal role of *Rhodiola rosea* in tipping the scale in the right direction.

Too Much Stress, Too Little Energy, Too Many Pounds

Chronic stress—and the anxiety, depression, and fatigue that often go along with it—factor heavily in overeating, particularly when we try to calm our nerves or boost our flagging energy with a favorite sweet or comfort food. We might get a quick lift from a chocolate bar or a cup of cappuccino, but once the effects wear off, we feel more drained than ever. Meanwhile, the number on the scale keeps inching higher.

This is because when we're chronically stressed, our adrenal glands release excess cortisol, which in turn causes fat to accumulate around our middles. Recent studies show that excess abdominal fat is a major risk factor for heart disease and diabetes.[5] It also is a sign of metabolic syndrome, an increasingly common by-product of a sedentary lifestyle.

In the United States, more than 40 million adults have metabolic syndrome, and the incidence among children and adolescents is on the rise.[6] Besides excess abdominal fat, markers for the condition include glucose intolerance, insulin resistance, abnormal lipid (LDL and HDL) levels, and disturbances in the hypothalamic-pituitary-adrenal axis. Not surprisingly, many of the same symptoms occur with chronic overactivation of the stress response system.[9]

Although careful eating and regular exercise are keys to weight loss and good health, those of us with excess pounds also must pay attention to stress, which often is at the root of weight problems. We already know that by strengthening the stress response system, *Rhodiola rosea* helps to reduce sensitivity to stress and to prevent the release of excess cortisol. So calming and balancing the stress response system may help to counteract the accumulation of abdominal fat, not to mention other aspects of metabolic syndrome.

In addition, by replenishing the body's energy reserves, *Rhodiola rosea* addresses three major contributors to weight gain: depression, anxiety, and low energy. It's no secret that when we're in a good mood, we're less likely to sit around consoling ourselves with Oreos. Likewise, once we shake free of persistent fatigue, not only do we feel more energized for exercise, we also are more motivated to eat healthfully and to take care of ourselves. Many of our patients who take *Rhodiola rosea* for depression, anxiety, or fatigue report a bonus benefit: As mood goes up, pounds go down.

FASTER FAT BURNING

Most of the fat that comes from our diets goes straight to adipose (fat) tissue, where it gets stored as triglycerides. In order to "burn fat," which releases energy to our cells, the body first must break down triglycerides into smaller free fatty acids—a process called lipolysis.

When certain enzymes, such as lipase, break down triglycerides, they send free fatty acids via the lymphatic and blood circulatory systems to cells throughout the body. Cells use these free fatty acids to produce energy in the mitochondria. Perilipins are proteins on the surface of fat droplets that prevent lipolytic enzymes from breaking down triglycerides. So anything that interferes with perilipin formation, including *Rhodiola rosea*, can speed up fat burning.

In animal studies, *Rhodiola rosea* increased the breakdown of triglycerides stored in fat tissue by stimulating lipolysis and reducing perilipins. This action helps speed up fat metabolism—and promotes weight loss in the process.[3, 4, 8] *Rhodiola rosea*'s balancing effect on the stress response system also helps to regulate fat metabolism. It works like this: The hypothalamic-pituitary-adrenal axis, a component of the stress response system, tends to function poorly when we're under chronic stress. This can disrupt the balance of fat metabolism and lipolysis, which in turn can lead to excess fat deposits around the waist.[7]

In other words, one reason that we gain weight when we're stressed-out is that the HPA axis isn't working properly. Conversely, excess weight prevents the HPA axis from doing its job as well as it could. So by stabilizing the HPA axis, *Rhodiola rosea* may help sustain normal lipolysis during times of stress—*and* keep us from putting on weight.

TWO HERBS
ARE BETTER THAN ONE

When weight loss is the primary goal, we seldom recommend *Rhodiola rosea* alone. It appears to work best when taken in tandem with another herb, *Rhododendron caucasicum*. This little-known species of rhododendron is native to the same regions as *Rhodiola rosea*. (Please do not eat the rhododendron that may be growing in your yard. It will make you *very* sick.)

Villagers living in the Altai and Caucasus mountains regularly combine *Rhodiola rosea* and *Rhododendron caucasicum*. The two herbs appear to work synergistically, each enhancing the effects of the other. Like *Rhodiola rosea*, *Rhododendron caucasicum* contains polyphenols, phenylpropanoids, and proanthocyanidins—all powerful antioxidants that help maintain cellular energy production and repair. As a bonus, *Rhododendron caucasicum* blocks the absorption of 20 percent of the fat from food when taken at the beginning of a meal.

Since the end of the Cold War, the problem of obesity has been getting more attention in Russia. In 1997, the Russian Ministry of Health sponsored a symposium called "Stress and Weight Management" as part of the national campaign "Russian Perestroika and Healthy Diet—97." At the symposium, Dr. Musa Abidoff, professor of medicine at the Moscow Center of Modern Medicine, presented the results of the first double-blind, placebo-controlled study to examine the effects of a product called Rhodalean-400—which contains

200 milligrams of *Rhodiola rosea* and 200 milligrams of *Rhododendron caucasicum* standardized extracts—on weight loss.

Dr. Abidoff's study involved 273 obese men and women, each with a body mass index between 29 and 34 kg/m^2. By comparison, the normal range for body mass index is between 18 and 25 kg/m^2. (*Kg* refers to a person's weight in kilograms, and *m* to height in meters.) All of the study participants were to limit their calorie intakes to 1,800 a day, and to walk for 20 minutes after lunch and dinner. In addition, half of the group took Rhodalean-400 three times a day, 30 minutes before meals. The rest took a placebo.

Of the 246 participants who completed the 20-week study, those using Rhodalean-400 got much better results, with a mean weight loss of 9.3 ± 1.4 kilograms. This translates to an average of 20.5 pounds, give or take 3.1 pounds. By comparison, those given the placebo tallied a mean weight loss of 1.2 ± 1.6 kilograms—an average of 2.6 pounds, give or take 3.5 pounds.

According to the study results, postmeal cortisol levels were 17 percent lower in the Rhodalean-400 group than in the placebo group. Perilipins were lower as well. Best of all, no side effects were reported.[2]

AN ANSWER TO THOSE POSTPREGNANCY POUNDS

Many women who gain weight during pregnancy and after childbirth struggle to get back to their prepregnancy size. A whole host of factors seems to conspire against weight loss, from the added stress of motherhood to hormonal changes, fatigue, lack of time for exercise, and constant exposure to kiddie foods.

Dr. Abidoff tested another formulation of Rhodalean—200

milligrams of *Rhodiola rosea* and 100 milligrams of *Rhododendron caucasicum*—in 45 women between ages 21 and 42 who weighed an average of 164.5 pounds. All of the women had given birth and had stopped lactating 4 months earlier. Their average obesity index was 130 percent, meaning that they were about 42 pounds above their ideal average weight of 126.5 pounds.

The women were to reduce their calorie intakes from 2,000 to between 1,750 and 1,850 by cutting back on carbohydrates and fat. They also were to eat the last meal of the day at least 3 hours before bedtime. After 6 weeks, the women taking Rhodalean had lost 5 to 6 percent of their weight, or roughly 8 to 10 pounds—compared with just 0.4 to 0.7 percent of body weight, or 0.7 to 1.1 pounds, for those taking a placebo. After 8 weeks, some had lost as much as 14 percent of their weight, or 23 pounds. The number on the scale continued to decline for another month. Even better, most of the pounds—11.5 percent, on average—seemed to come from the waist area, a strategic location for good health.[1] Among those in the placebo group, only 1.7 to 2.2 percent of the weight loss was from the waist.

Dr. Abidoff's findings are consistent with our own clinical experience. Patients whose weight gain results from anxiety, depression, stress, or fatigue, and who are willing to walk for 20 minutes twice a day, successfully slim down once they add *Rhodiola rosea* to their treatment regimens. For patients whose excess weight is a primary health concern, the two-herbs-plus-exercise approach produces excellent results.

How to take *Rhodiola rosea* . . .

To Achieve a Healthy Weight

The most effective way to lose weight and trim the gut is to combine Rhodiola rosea *and* Rhododendron caucasicum *with moderate daily exercise and moderate calorie restriction—between 1,700 and 1,800 calories a day, on average. People who are small in build may need to cut back even more, to 1,500 calories a day, while those who are larger or more physically active may be able to eat between 1,900 and 2,000 calories a day. Of course, if you stick with this regimen for 4 weeks and you don't see any change on the scale, then you should reduce your daily calorie intake or increase your daily walking time until you see results.*

While the herbal formulas used in Dr. Abidoff's studies combine Rhodiola rosea *and* Rhododendron caucasicum, *we recommend separate herbal supplements. This is because* Rhodiola rosea *is best absorbed when taken 20 to 30 minutes before a meal, while* Rhododendron caucasicum *reduces fat absorption most effectively when taken right at the beginning of a meal.*

Start with 200 milligrams of Rhodiola rosea *½ hour before breakfast and ½ hour before lunch—a total of 400 milligrams a day—for an optimal daytime energy boost. Add 100 to 200 milligrams of* Rhododendron caucasicum *right before breakfast, lunch, and/or dinner. If you need a simpler regimen, you can take both supplements at the same time before breakfast and lunch.*

PART III

ENERGIZED

FOR LIFE

CHAPTER 15

The
BUILDING
BLOCKS
OF ENERGY

Rhodiola rosea increases energy within cells and supports the optimal function of virtually every system in the body. But it can't do the job alone. A single herb can't completely wipe out the effects of too much stress or too little sleep. No matter how potent or beneficial, it can't make up for a diet that lacks energizing foods. Nor can it compensate for the weight gain and sluggishness that often accompany a sedentary lifestyle. No such magic pill exists, in either conventional or alternative medicine.

The challenge of maximizing energy rests on our own shoulders. The good news is, we can do much to replenish and sustain our energy reserves and to improve our odds of living well. Taking *Rhodiola rosea* is one important strategy. In this chapter, we'll explore the rest.

The High-Energy Diet

Food provides the fuel that your body needs to produce energy. The number of calories in a food is a measure of its energy content. The more calories you take in, the more *potential* energy you have.

But while food is your body's primary energy source, eating too much actually can leave you feeling less energetic. So why doesn't pigging out solve your body's energy crisis? The answers are simple. First, your body needs its energy in a steady stream, not in peaks and valleys. Second, it depends on foods rich in key vitamins, minerals, and other nutrients—not those rich in calories—to support essential functions such as producing cellular energy, building cell components, and supporting cellular defense and repair mechanisms. Third, when you take in more calories than your body can use, the excess gets stored as fat. This fat provides energy only if you burn it, not if it sits in storage around your waist.

The ideal diet features a variety of foods that provide just the right number of calories to meet your body's basic energy requirements and all of the necessary nutrients to maintain cellular energy production. We suggest a diet that supplies about 1,800 calories a day. This figure is based on the typical calorie needs of a 150-pound person. Naturally, you should adjust the figure for your size—1,500 calories if you're under 125 pounds, 2,000 calories if you're over 175 pounds.

You also need to consider your activity level. People with high-intensity exercise programs and those with physically demanding jobs require extra calories and protein. On the other hand, those with sedentary jobs must not only watch their calorie intakes but also stay as active as possible during their leisure time in order to avoid weight gain.

The good news is that following a high-energy diet is a sensible way to achieve and maintain a healthy weight. Just adopt these eight nutritional principles, and you will feel—and see—the difference.

Build each meal around a palm-size serving of low-fat protein. Good sources include soy, fish, skinless chicken, and egg whites. In general, try to limit red meat to no more than four servings a month. If you're following a vegetarian diet, be sure to eat combinations of whole grains, beans (including soy and soy products), nuts and seeds, and dairy products. This way, you'll get a full complement of essential amino acids—the building blocks of protein—at every meal. Vegetarians also should take 1,000 micrograms of vitamin B_{12} every day.

Aim for four or five servings of fruits and at least four servings of vegetables every day—and the more, the better. Fruits and vegetables provide the vitamins, minerals, and antioxidants that prevent free radical damage to cells and support the repair mechanisms vital to cellular energy production. To get the most energy and nutrients, whenever possible choose fruits and vegetables that are grown locally, in season, and certified organic. Choose a variety of colors, too. The reason: Different colors suggest different nutritional compositions, and you want to be sure that you're getting the best mix of nutrients you can. For fruits, one serving equals ½ cup of berries or a medium-size fruit; for veggies, one serving equals 1 cup of leafy greens or ½ cup of a nonleafy vegetable.

Save room for five servings of whole grains a day. Whole grains supply slow-burning carbohydrates, which the body digests and metabolizes over many hours to release their energy. In contrast, carbs from refined grains such as white flour and white rice are processed much more quickly. This is bad news for the body's energy supply.

Your best bet is to limit candies, cookies, pastries, snack foods, white bread, crackers, pastas, and—sad to say—bagels, replacing them with whole grain breads, brown rice, quinoa, oats, and barley.

Besides providing a more constant level of energy than refined grains, whole grains deliver many more vitamins and minerals, plus the fiber that's so important for reducing the risk of cardiovascular disease and cancer. One serving of whole grains equals one slice of bread, ½ cup of dry cereal, or ½ cup of cooked rice, pasta, or cooked cereal.

Think three for beans, nuts, and seeds. Three servings per day, that is. A serving equals ½ cup of cooked beans; 2 tablespoons of sunflower, sesame, or pumpkin seeds; 2 tablespoons of almond butter; or ⅓ cup of nuts.

Beans are an excellent source of protein, not to mention slow-burning carbohydrates. You have a wide variety to choose from. Look in your supermarket for kidney, cannelini, lima, mung, red, soy, adzuki, black, pinto, and navy beans, as well as lentils, chickpeas, and pigeon peas.

As for nuts, research has shown that they can help prevent cardio-vascular disease. The most healthful are walnuts and almonds because they derive fewer calories from fat than other nuts and they supply lots of vitamins and minerals. By comparison, Brazil nuts, pecans, and pistachios are high in fat. Cashews, macadamias, and pignoli (pine nuts) are even worse. Eat them only on occasion, and only in very small amounts.

Don't forget flaxseeds, which when ground up are a wonderful source of omega-3 essential fatty acids. And sesame seeds contain less common amino acids that help to round out and complete the proteins from other foods.

Get enough dairy on a daily basis. Aim for one or two servings of low-fat or fat-free dairy products every day. Your best bets include 1 cup of low-fat or fat-free yogurt, ½ cup of low-fat cottage cheese, 1 cup of low-fat or fat-free milk, and 1 ounce of reduced-fat or low-fat cheese such as part-skim mozzarella or feta.

Among fats, separate the good from the bad and the ugly. The good fats contain mono- and polyunsaturated fatty acids, which tend to increase "good" HDL cholesterol and decrease "bad" LDL cholesterol. Examples of these beneficial fats include olive, canola, soy, sunflower, safflower, and flaxseed oils. You can have up to 1 tablespoon of an unsaturated oil once a day (or 1 teaspoon three times a day). Use the oil to sauté vegetables or to make salad dressing. Never heat flaxseed oil, though, because it destroys the omega-3 essential fatty acids.

Bad fats are saturated fats, the kind found in red meat, pork, bacon, duck and other fatty poultry, chicken fat, and lard, as well as whole milk, cheese, butter, and ice cream. Also avoid oils that are solid at room temperature, such as palm and coconut, and those that are made from lard and other animal fats. These are high in saturated fat, too.

By far the worst are the trans fats, which occur as byproducts of the manufacturing process that converts liquid oils into solid fats such as stick margarine and shortening. Unfortunately, trans fats are everywhere, including commercial desserts and most of the menu items served by fast food chains. If the ingredient list of a particular food refers to "partially hydrogenated" anything, that means trans fats.

Use spices with abandon. Spices are the best way to add flavor and variety to your diet without extra calories. Many spices offer health benefits of their own, and have long histories as folk remedies. For example, garlic, ginger, and Indian spices such as coriander and turmeric are known to supply nutrients and antioxidants that support cellular energy production as well as the cells' defense and repair mechanisms. So trade in your saltshaker for these, as well as for sprinkles of cinnamon, nutmeg, black peppercorns, fennel, cloves, mustard seeds, curry, saffron, cumin, and caraway. For a dash of extra nutrition, try seasoning your cooking with fresh basil, cilantro, bay leaves, parsley, or mint.

Stay well hydrated. This means drinking at least six glasses of water per day.

ESSENTIAL HERBAL AND NUTRITIONAL SUPPLEMENTS

Nutritional supplements can help us maintain our energy and reduce our chances of getting sick. The fact is, as hard as we may try, most of us don't get all of the vitamins, minerals, and antioxidants we need from the foods we eat. Taking supplements can help ensure that our bodies get a full complement of essential nutrients.

Rather than advising our patients to down handfuls of pills every day, we offer the following basic supplement regimen. This is by no means a comprehensive list, just our top five picks—in addition to *Rhodiola rosea*, of course.

Multivitamin: A good multivitamin/mineral supplement supplies nearly 100 percent of the Daily Value for each essential vitamin and mineral.

Vitamin B-complex: Taking more than the Daily Values for the B vitamins is like supplemental health insurance. It helps to maintain and improve the function of every cell in your body, especially those in your brain.[2] You can purchase an inexpensive B-complex such as B50 or B100, or you can splurge on the Rolls Royce of B vitamins—Bio-strath, a Swiss preparation that also is rich in antioxidants.

Antioxidants: Now that you know how oxygen free radicals can damage cells and deplete your energy supply, you probably want to add antioxidants to your supplement regimen. Because there are many kinds of free radicals, we recommend getting many kinds of antioxidants in supplement form, in addition to eating antioxidant-rich fruits and vegetables. See page 229 for a consumer's guide to high-quality antioxidant products.

SAM-e: By the time you turn 40, you need extra nutrients to preserve healthy brain function. *Rhodiola rosea* tops the list, followed by

SAM-e. Short for S-adenosylmethionine, SAM-e is a natural metabolite that contributes to more than 100 biochemical reactions in every cell of the body. It also supports the production of essential neurotransmitters, proteins, and antioxidants; maintains cellular energy; protects against oxidative (free radical) damage; and repairs damaged cells.

Research has shown that SAM-e is a highly effective treatment for depression, as well as for arthritis and liver disease. Still, people with bipolar disorder should check with their doctors before taking SAM-e. Because it's an antidepressant, it can trigger manic symptoms.

Most SAM-e products have not received adequate testing for quality and shelf life. If not properly manufactured, they can deteriorate rapidly. Be sure to check page 230 for some reliable SAM-e brands before buying.

Omega-3 essential fatty acids: These beneficial fats maintain the fluidity of nerve cell membranes. They also are important for building cells; for preserving brain, nerve, and eye function; and for lowering the risk of high cholesterol, cardiovascular disease, and cancer. We recommend taking 1,000 to 3,000 milligrams of omega-3s in supplement form every day. Be sure to refrigerate after opening.

ACTIVE BODY, ENGAGED MIND

Being active is one of the best ways to build up our energy reserves. But despite the proven health benefits of physical activity, people are more sedentary than ever. Ironically, many say that they don't exercise because they lack the energy for it. If you're one of them, here's how to switch into fitness mode.

First, review the list of energy enhancers and energy drains in chapter 3, and think about what you can do to maximize the former and eliminate the latter. This alone may provide enough "juice" to increase your level of physical activity.

Next, you need to find time—or create time—in your schedule for workouts. For example, after dinner, your instinct may be to flop in your favorite chair and flip on the TV. Instead, slip on your sneakers and stroll to the end of your driveway. Once you're in the fresh air, you may feel the urge to walk farther. Alternatively, you could turn off the TV and go to bed, so you wake up early enough to squeeze in 30 minutes on the treadmill.

EXERCISE AND THE STRESS RESPONSE

Our bodies are best able to adapt to the physical stress of exercise when we work out regularly, increase our capacity slowly, and alternate periods of activity with intervals of recovery. We can support this process by taking *Rhodiola rosea*, which is proven to help build physical strength and endurance. (To learn more, see chapter 7.)

In general, the more demanding an activity is, the more free radicals it produces. The good news is that over time, regular workouts help the body adapt to the stepped-up release of free radicals by increasing antioxidants and cellular repair components. In the long run, this reduces free radical damage and improves resistance to future oxidative stress.[4] The key—as with most things in life—is *moderation*.

30 MINUTES WILL DO

You don't need much exercise to reap its energy- and health-enhancing benefits. Studies show that 30 minutes of moderate-intensity physical activity every day can substantially improve your health. Burning 1,000 calories per week through exercise seems to be the minimum for reducing the risk of age-related illnesses such as heart disease, colon cancer, and diabetes.[1, 3]

If you don't have the time or inclination to do traditional structured workouts such as aerobics, jogging, or treadmill, you can get similar health benefits from everyday lifestyle activities.[3] For example, housework, yard work, or active play with children is as effective as calisthenics when done at an intensity comparable to brisk walking.

MENTAL AEROBICS

The adage "use it or lose it" applies as much to our brains as to our bodies. The more active our minds are, the more mental energy we have. This is true even as we get older. In fact, scientists are discovering that many of the supposed age-related changes that affect the mind—especially memory loss—have more to do with mental activity and engagement than with age. For example, Stanford University researchers have found that we can improve our memory skills by 30 to 50 percent simply by practicing mental exercises on a regular basis.

There are as many ways to stimulate our brains as we can dream up. Some ideas:

• Reading newspapers, magazines, and books

• Doing crossword puzzles

• Playing "thinking" games such as Scrabble, charades, chess, checkers, bridge, backgammon, and Trivial Pursuit

• Taking a course at a local college or studying a foreign language

• Learning to play a musical instrument

• Adopting a new hobby, such as painting, writing, photography, or woodworking

THE ENERGIZING EFFECTS
OF GOOD COMPANY

Strong connections to family, friends, and the larger community in which we live help to keep us mentally sharp and physically energized. In contrast, the perception of being alone—of having no one else to count on—can be exceptionally stressful. People who experience this sort of isolation can feel vulnerable and anxious, especially when something goes wrong. Then their minds latch on to all kinds of worries, activating the stress response system and draining away energy.

The most potent antidote to the stress of social isolation, of course, is social connection. Bonding and belonging, loving and being loved help to calm the stress response system. In this way, positive social interactions can be soothing and energizing at the same time.

GETTING CONNECTED

By tracking social networks in large populations, researchers have confirmed what members of tight-knit communities around the world know intuitively: We *need* one another, not just for physical survival but for emotional and spiritual well-being, too.

So what do we make of such findings? Should we become more active at church, volunteer at a soup kitchen, join a bridge game, or check out one of those online matchmaking services? The answer may be yes—or no—to all of the above. Just as an exercise program needs to be tailored to individual temperament, the same commonsense wisdom applies to a social network.

For some people, close relationships with family and friends provide a strong enough sense of belonging. For others, being an active member of a church, synagogue, temple, mosque, or another spiritual community buoys the mind and spirit. Volunteering to help others appears to have positive health benefits. The point is, do what feels most authentic for *you*.

Though close relationships stimulate and nourish us in so many ways, they can deplete us of vital energy when they're unbalanced. Friends or family members who talk but don't listen, who take but don't give, who expect us to help with their problems but don't reciprocate drain our emotional reservoirs. We may need to limit the amount of energy we invest in such unhealthy relationships.

SLEEP AND OTHER NATURAL RHYTHMS

Shakespeare described sleep as "Nature's soft nurse." In truth, sleep is as essential to our well-being as the food we eat. While we sleep, complex biochemical processes replenish our energy reserves and repair damaged cells and tissues throughout the body.

Adults need somewhere between 7 and 8 hours of sleep during every 24-hour period. When we don't get enough rest, we not only jeopardize our mental and physical performance, but we also increase our risk of weakened immune function, type 2 diabetes, and obesity. Sleep deprivation is emotionally taxing, too. We're more prone to stress, anxiety, anger, and sadness when we don't get enough sleep. With all the demands and temptations of our wired world, most of us are struggling not to build up a large sleep debt. And in children, even mild sleep disruption can seriously interfere with cognitive development and learning ability.[5]

So what can we do to safeguard our sleep? Anyone who suffers from chronic insomnia, sleep apnea, or another sleep disorder may require medical treatment. Most of us, though, can benefit from these commonsense self-care guidelines.

- Keep regular hours as much as possible. Try to go to bed at the same time every night and wake up at the same time every morning. And try not to sleep more than 2 hours later than usual on weekends.

- Adopt a bedtime routine to help prepare your mind and body for sleep. It might include a hot bath, a cup of soothing herbal tea, or a relaxation practice. Reading in bed is okay, too—but choose calming reading material and be sure to avoid bright light.

- Eat your evening meal at least 3 hours before retiring for the night. And avoid stimulants—including chocolate and caffeinated sodas, teas, and coffee—after 5:00 P.M.

- Do not drink alcohol right before bed. Although a "nightcap" may help you fall asleep, you could wake up once the effects wear off, a phenomenon known as rebound insomnia.

- Plan your workouts for at least 3 hours before bedtime. Exercising during the day—especially in the late afternoon or early evening—can help train your brain to follow the right pattern of sleep and wakefulness. On the other hand, if you exercise within 3 hours of going to bed, your body won't have enough time to settle down for sleep.

- Create an inviting sleep environment. Make sure that the room temperature, mattresses, sheets, and covers are comfortable for you.

- If you have a television or computer in your bedroom, move it elsewhere. Use your bedroom almost exclusively for sleep.

Naps of 30 to 40 minutes in length can be an excellent source of energy renewal when normal sleep is not possible. But beware: Naps of longer duration may lead to deeper sleep, so you wake up feeling groggy and fatigued, instead of rested and refreshed.

RENEWAL THROUGH RITUAL AND ROUTINE

Rituals and routines allow us to tune in to the rhythms of our bodies and the world around us. Many social traditions connect us to the natural cycles of life and the changes of the seasons. In traditional societies, regular shared meals and holidays among extended families, observance of community and religious festivals, coming together in groups to play music and dance—all serve to bolster each person's sense of belonging and to reduce stress and replenish energy.

Daily routines have the same beneficial effect as more formal, symbolic rituals. They calm us because we know what to expect. Although at times our routines may make life seem too predictable, they also provide a solid foundation—a "holding environment," in the words of British psychoanalyst D. W. Winnicott[6]—that restores and sustains us as we take on the challenges of an ever-changing world.

We have many opportunities to create routines in our lives. Among the possibilities are exercise programs, team sports, family game nights, visits to relatives, regular uninterrupted "quiet times," repeat trips to favorite destinations, monthly dinners, and book clubs. In short, anything that we can count on becomes part of our foundation, our personal "holding environment."

HARNESSING ENERGY FROM WITHIN

There's one more essential energy source that we need to consider, and that is a calm, clear mind. Maintaining a healthy mindset can have a profound and positive influence on our energy levels.

The gateway to a calm, clear mind is the present moment. When we're in the present, we understand that whatever is happening is inevitable. We don't waste vital energy getting trapped in negative thought loops about the past or the future. We stop trying to change what we cannot. By the same token, we see more clearly what we *can* change, and with this awareness we can use our energy more productively. When we let go of our preconceived notions and expectations about how things ought to be, we can embrace each moment as it unfolds, instead of wallowing in disappointment.

Yet while we may understand this and even agree to it in principle, it runs counter to the way in which our minds are conditioned to work. This is why for most of us understanding by itself isn't enough. We need tools to experience the present moment. Fortunately, every spiritual tradition has practices that can help us. They include singing and chanting, meditation and prayer, yoga and tai chi, and deep breathing.

HEALING IN THE HERE AND NOW

Dick's alertness to the present moment drew his attention to the practice that has helped both of us to optimize our energy, mental clarity, and happiness.

Dick: In 1990, I was invited to give a lecture on herbal treatments for depression at a United Nations conference. Another speaker at the meeting—which was held in a stiflingly hot room—was a woman who teaches a form of yogic breathing called Sudarshan Kriya Yoga

(SKY). Breathing courses based on SKY are sponsored by the Art of Living Foundation, a nonprofit organization that does charitable and relief work in more than 100 countries.

The woman's presentation made a strong impression on me. I had tried many breathing techniques over the years—I had even been cured of hepatitis after practicing an intensive Japanese-style purification technique—so I thought I knew a lot about them. But I was struck by the fact that in such an incredibly hot room, everyone was soaked in sweat—everyone, that is, except the speaker and another teacher from the Art of Living Foundation, who was 9 months pregnant. They were the only people who appeared to be completely relaxed and comfortable.

Although I didn't think I needed another spiritual practice in addition to Zen and aikido, I was so impressed with what I saw and heard that day that I began recommending the SKY breathing course to patients struggling with stress, anxiety, depression, and post-traumatic stress disorder. Much to my delight, the course turned out to be so effective that some of my patients were able to reduce their reliance on medications. Many others reported unexpected health benefits—increases in their physical and mental energy, as well as improvements in medical conditions and relief from chronic pain.

I decided to sign up for a SKY breathing course myself. And I convinced Pat, who was rather skeptical, to join me.

Pat: I had never been able to sit still or quiet my mind long enough to meditate. Even though I'm trained in hypnosis and I've benefited from guided imagery, the thought of committing 20 precious minutes every day to just sitting and breathing—especially when I had so much to do—was totally unappealing. At the same time, even though *Rhodiola rosea* had dramatically improved my energy and endurance after my bout with Lyme disease, I wasn't 100 percent better. So finally I agreed to take the SKY breathing course with Dick.

On the first night of the course, I was sure that I had made a big mistake. The teachings seemed elementary, and I felt angry. But once we advanced to the deepest level of breathing, everything changed for me. The stress that had built up over years of my being ill finally left my system. I felt a tremendous sense of relief and lightness.

Since that weekend, my breathing practice—combined with yoga, meditation, daily walks, and *Rhodiola rosea*—have continued to improve my health and well-being and have helped me to become pain-free. Dick's response was equally profound.

Dick: Even though I had been through years of meditation and breathing practice, with the SKY technique I experienced the complete unification of mind, body, and spirit. I felt a bottomless ocean of joy open inside me.

EVERY BREATH YOU TAKE

Soon after completing the SKY breathing course, we began to research how breathing affects the nervous system. We discovered that voluntary control of breathing patterns activates and tones the parasympathetic nervous system. As it turns out, the lungs have thousands of receptors that send messages through the vagus nerve to the cerebral cortex and emotional control centers of the brain. It is the vagus nerve, in concert with the hypothalamus, that stimulates the release of hormones not only to help protect against stress but also to increase our sense of connectedness to others and to the world around us.[2]

In light of all this, it isn't surprising that when we practice the SKY technique, we can feel how yoga breathing boosts our energy supply and balances the stress response system—much as *Rhodiola rosea* does.[2] In fact, both *Rhodiola rosea* and yoga breathing have the dual effect of producing a state of alertness, along with a calm, clear mind.

Live in the Present Moment

By shining the light of awareness on your experience at any given moment, you can disengage from repetitive, negative thoughts and emotions and free up precious energy. Joy is available to you right now, at this very moment. As our dear friend Dr. Beth Abrams wrote during the Art of Living course:

> *The reed that sways in the breeze,*
> *Hollow and empty*
> *Is a timeless flute through which*
> *Infinite Breath*
> *Plays a song in my heart.*

—*Grace Notes*, July 26, 2003

For More Information

Organizations

American Botanical Council
512-926-4900
www.herbalgram.org
A nonprofit organization committed to providing unbiased scientific information on the medicinal properties and uses of plants.

Herb Research Foundation
303-449-2265
www.herbs.org
Founded by Andrew Weil in coordination with the American Botanical Council; publishes *Herbalgram*, a journal that reviews herbs and features abstracts of recent studies in scientific journals. Offers monographs of herbs for a small fee.

National Center for Complementary and Alternative Medicine (NCCAM)
888-644-6226
www.nccam.nih.gov
Provides updates on ongoing research trials involving herbs. (Call the toll-free number for the NCCAM Clearinghouse, which can answer questions about complementary and alternative medicine.)

Natural Medicines Comprehensive Database
209-472-2244
www.naturaldatabase.com
Covers all of the common and many of the less well-known herbs. Includes information on side effects and potential drug interactions.

Print Resources

Brown, Richard P., Patricia L. Gerbarg, and Phillip R. Muskin. "Complementary and Alternative Treatments in Psychiatry." In *Psychiatry* 2nd edition. Edited by Allan Tasman, Jerald Kay, and Jeffrey Lieberman. Hoboken, NJ: Wiley, 2003.
Discusses a broad range of herbs and supplements, as well as medications commonly used in other countries.

227

Ernst, Edzard, ed. *The Desktop Guide to Complementary and Alternative Medicine: An Evidence-Based Approach.* St. Louis, MO: Mosby, 2001.
A well-organized and well-documented resource for the clinical applications and side effects of commonly used herbs.

Robbers, James, and Varro Tyler. *Tyler's Herbs of Choice.* Binghamton, NY: Hawthorne Herbal Press, 1999.
An excellent, consumer-friendly review of common herbal remedies for various medical conditions.

WEB SITES

www.artofliving.org
Provides information on Sudarshan Kriya yoga and includes yoga breathing courses available throughout the United States and the world.

www.consumerlab.com
Regularly updates its independent evaluations of many supplement brands.

www.fda.gov/medwatch
www.cfsan.fda.gov/~dms/supplmnt.html
Lists recalls and warnings about poor-quality or unsafe brands.

www.hmrprogram.com
Offers a complete weight-loss program combining diet, supplements, mild exercise, and nutritional counseling through hospitals and clinics. (For a telephone version of the program, visit www.hmrathome.com.)

www.ornish.com
Sound dietary advice, especially for heart health.

www.rhodiolarosea.org
An excellent source of information and research on *Rhodiola rosea.*

www.supplementwatch.com
Provides good overviews and independent ratings of the quality, safety, and value of supplement products.

www.weightwatchers.com
The official Web site for Weight Watchers, which now offers FlexPoints, a weight-loss program that assigns point values to foods.

Buying Quality Herbs and Supplements

You can find many of the following products in drugstores and health food stores. While we feel comfortable recommending them, be aware that manufacturers sometimes change their formulations. For this reason, we suggest periodically rechecking product quality and content—perhaps through one of the consumer Web sites on the opposite page.

Herb/ Nutrient	Manufacturer/ Brand	Contact Information
Antioxidants	Himalaya/Geriforte	www.himalaya-proselect.com
Astragalus	Nature's Way Nature's Herbs	www.naturesway.com www.herbalvillage.com
B vitamins	Nature's Answer/Bio-Strath	800-439-2324 www.naturesanswer.com
Cat's claw (Saventaro)	Medicine Plants Phytopharmica	www.medicine-plants.com www.phytopharmica.com
Clear Mind	Ameriden International	www.ameriden.com
Cordyceps sinensis	New Chapter Pharmanex	www.new-chapter.com www.pharmanex.com
Eleutherococcus senticosus (Siberian ginseng)	Hsu's Ginseng	800-826-1577 www.hsuginseng,com
GalantaMind	Smart Nutrition	www.smart-nutrition.net
Galantamine/Rhodiola rosea	Ameriden International/ A/P Formula	www.ameriden.com
Ginkgo	Nature's Way/Ginkgold Pharmaton/Ginkoba	www.naturesway.com www.pharmaton.com
Ginseng (Panax)	Hsu's Ginseng	800-826-1577 www.hsuginseng.com

Herb/ Nutrient	Manufacturer/ Brand	Contact Information
Maca	Medicine Plants/MACA750	800-584-0228 www.medicine-plants.com
Omega-3 fatty acids	Solgar, Schiff, Natrol, Twin Labs	Available in health food stores
Optygen	First Endurance	www.firstendurance.com
Piracetam/aniracetam	International Antiaging Systems (IAS)	www.antiaging-systems.com
Prime 1	Advantage Marketing Systems	www.oak-tree.org/ams-products.html
Rhodiola rosea		
100 mg capsules (1% salidrosides/3% rosavins)	Ameriden International	www.ameriden.com
170 mg capsules (1% salidrosides/3% rosavins)	Bodyonics Pinnacle Rhodax	GNC (General Nutrition Centers) www.gnc.com
180 mg tablets (2% salidrosides/4% rosavins)	Kare-N-Herbs/Energy Care	www.kare-n-herbs.com
Rhododendron caucasicm	Ameriden International	www.ameriden.com
SAM-e	Nature Made/SAM-e	800-276-2878 www.naturemade.com
	IAS/Donamet or SAMYR	www.antiaging-systems.com
Schizandra chinesis	Kare-N-Herbs	www.kare-n-herbs.com
Second Wind	Botanica Bioscience	www.botanica-bioscience.com
Shark liver oil	Smart Nutrition/Izami Lane Laboratory/Immunofin Life Extension Foundation	www.smart-nutrition.com www.lanelabs.com www.lef.com
Synergy	Ameriden International	www.ameriden.com
Withania somnifera	Himalaya USA	800-869-4640 www.himalayausa.com
	Ayurceutics	www.ayurceutics.com

References

Chapter 1

1. Franceschi, C., et al., "The Network and the Remodeling Theories of Aging: Historical Background and New Perspectives," *Experimental Gerontology* 35, no. 6–7 (2000): 879–96.

2. Kessler, R. C., et al., "The Epidemiology of Major Depressive Disorder: Results from the National Comorbidity Survey Replication (NCS-R)," *JAMA: The Journal of the American Medical Association* 289, no. 23 (2003): 3095–3105.

3. Perls, T., "Genetic and Environmental Influences on Exceptional Longevity and the AGE Nomogram," *Annals of the New York Academy of Sciences* 959 (2002): 1–13.

4. Sastre, J., et al., "Mitochondrial Damage in Aging and Apoptosis," *Annals of the New York Academy of Sciences* 959 (2002): 448–51.

5. Selye, H., "Studies on Adaptation," *Endocrinology*, no. 21 (1937): 169–88.

6. Singh, R. B., et al., "Brain-Heart Connection and the Risk of Heart Attack," *Biomedicine and Pharmacotherapy* 56, suppl. no. 2 (2002): S257–S265.

7. Tritschler, H. J., L. Packer, and R. Medori, "Oxidative Stress and Mitochondrial Dysfunction in Neurodegeneration," *Biochemistry and Molecular Biology International* 34, no. 1 (1994): 169–81.

Chapter 2

1. Aron, E. N., *The Highly Sensitive Person* (New York: Broadway Books, 1997).

2. Beauchaine, T., "Vagal Tone, Development, and Gray's Motivational Theory: Toward an Integrated Model of Autonomic Nervous System Functioning in Psychopathology," *Development and Psychopathology* 13, no. 2 (2001): 183–214.

3. Butler, R. N., et al., "Is There an Antiaging Medicine?" *Journals of Gerontology. Series A, Biological Sciences and Medical Sciences* 57A, no. 9 (2002): B_33–B338.

4. Carney, R. M., et al., "Association of Depression with Reduced Heart Rate Variability in Coronary Artery Disease," *American Journal of Cardiology* 76, no. 8 (1995): 562–64.

5. Carney, R. M., et al., "The Relationship between Heart Rate, Heart Rate Variability and Depression in Patients with Coronary Artery Disease," *Journal of Psychosomatic Research* 32, no. 2 (1988): 159–64.

6. Fabes, R. A., et al., "The Relations of Children's Emotion Regulation to Their Vicarious Emotional Responses and Comforting Behaviors," *Child Development* 65, no. 6 (1994): 1678–93.

7. Franceschi, C., et al., "The Network and the Remodeling Theories of Aging: Historical Background and New Perspectives," *Experimental Gerontology* 35, no. 6–7 (2000): 879–96.

8. Friedman, B. H., and J. F. Thayer, "Anxiety and Autonomic Flexibility: A Cardiovascular Approach," *Biological Psychiatry* 47, no. 3 (1998): 243–63.

9. Friedman, B. H., and J. F. Thayer, "Autonomic Balance Revisited: Panic Anxiety and Heart Rate Variability," *Journal of Psychosomatic Research* 44, no. 1 (1998): 133–51.

10. Goleman, D., narrator, *Destructive Emotions: A Scientific Dialogue with the Dalai Lama* (New York: Bantam Books, 2003).

11. Habib, K. E., P. W. Gold, and G. P. Chrousos, "Neuroendocrinology of Stress," *Neuroendocrinology* 30, no. 3 (2001): 695–728.

12. Mattson, M. P., W. Duan, and Z. Guo, "Meal Size and Frequency Affect Neuronal Plasticity and Vulnerability to Disease: Cellular and Molecular Mechanisms," *Journal of Neurochemistry* 84, no. 3 (2003): 417–31.

13. Mezzacappa, E., et al., "Anxiety, Antisocial Behavior, and Heart Rate Regulation in Adolescent Males," *Journal of Child Psychology and Psychiatry, and Allied Disciplines* 38, no. 4 (1997): 457–69.

14. Mezzacappa, E., et al., "Relationship of Aggression and Anxiety to Autonomic Regulation of Heart Rate Variability in Adolescent Males," *Annals of the New York Academy of Sciences* 794 (1996): 376–79.

15. Porges, S. W., "The Polyvagal Theory: Phylogenetic Substrates of a Social Nervous System," *International Journal of Psychophysiology* 42, no. 2 (2001): 123–46.

16. Porges, S. W., "The Vagus: A Mediator of Behavioral and Visceral Features Associated with Autism," in *The Neurobiology of Autism*, eds. M. L. Bauman and T. L. Kemper (Baltimore: Johns Hopkins University Press, 2004).

17. Rozman, K. K., and J. Doull, "Scientific Foundations of Hormesis: Maturation, Strengths, Limitations, and Possible Applications in Toxicology, Pharmacology, and Epidemiology," pt. 2, *Critical Reviews in Toxicology* 33, no. 3–4 (2003): 451–62.

18. Sahar, T., A. Y. Shalev, and S. W. Porges, "Vagal Modulation of Responses to Mental Challenge in Posttraumatic Stress Disorder," *Biological Psychiatry* 49, no. 7 (2001): 637–43.

19. Selye, H., "Studies on Adaptation," *Endocrinology*, no. 21 (1937): 169–88.

20. Thayer, J. F., B. H. Friedman, and T. D. Borkovec, "Autonomic Characteristics of Generalized Anxiety Disorder and Worry," *Biological Psychiatry* 39, no. 4 (1996): 255–66.

21. Tsigos, C., and G. P. Chrousos, "Hypothalamic-Pituitary-Adrenal Axis, Neuroendocrine Factors and Stress," *Journal of Psychosomatic Research* 53, no. 4 (2002): 865–71.

22. Winnicott, D. W., "The Theory of the Parent-Infant Relationship," *International Journal of Psycho-Analysis* 43 (1962): 238–39.

CHAPTER 4

1. Abidoff, M., et al. "*Rhodiola rosea* root extracrt Rhodax reduces inflammatory plasma C-reactive protein and creatine kinase in healthy volunteers. a placebo-controlled, double-blind clinical trial." *Experimental Biology and Medicine* in press (2004).

2. Abidoff, M. T., "Synergistic Effect of *Rhodiola Rosea* and *Rhododendron Caucasicum* Herbal Supplement on Weight Loss in Healthy Female Volunteers: Placebo Controlled Clinical Study" (forthcoming), in Russian, Grant 77–1997, Moscow, 1997.

3. *Apollonius of Rhodes: Jason and the Golden Fleece*, trans. R. Hunter, Oxford World's Classics (Oxford: Oxford University Press, 1998).

4. Baranov, V. B., "The Response of Cardiovascular System to Dosed Physical Load under the Effect of Herbal Adaptogen," in Russian, Contract 93-11-615, Phase I and Phase II, Moscow, Russian Federation Ministry of Health Institute of Medical and Biological Problems (IMBP), 1994.

5. Bespalov, V. G., et al., "The Inhibiting Effect of Phytoadaptogenic Preparations from Bioginseng, Eleutherococcus Senticosus *and* Rhaponticum Carthamoides *on the Development of Nervous System Tumors in Rats Induced by N-Nitrosoethylurea," in Russian,* Voprosy Onkologii 38, no. 9 (1992): 1073–80.

6. Bhattacharya, A., S. Ghosal, and S. K. Bhattacharya, "Anti-Oxidant Effect of Withania Somnifera Glycowithanolides in Chronic Footshock Stress-Induced Perturbations of Oxidative Free Radical Scavenging Enzymes and Lipid Peroxidation in Rat Frontal Cortex and Striatum," *Journal of Ethnopharmacology* 74, no. 1 (2001): 1–6.

7. Bhattacharya, S. K., and A. V. Muruganandam, "Adaptogenic Activity of Withania Somnifera: An Experimental Study Using a Rat Model of Chronic Stress," *Pharmacology, Biochemistry, and Behavior* 75, no. 3 (2003): 547–55.

8. Brekhman, I. I., and I. V. Dardymov, "New Substances of Plant Origin Which Increase Non-Specific Resistance," *Annual Review of Pharmacology*, no. 9 (1968): 419–30.

9. Brown, R. P., P. G. Gerbarg, and Z. Ramazanov, "*Rhodiola Rosea:* A Phytomedical Review," *HerbalGram*, no. 56 (2002): 41–52.

10. Bucci, L. R., "Selected Herbals and Human Exercise Performance," *American Journal of Clinical Nutrition* 72, suppl. no. 2 (2000): S624–S636.

11. Davydov, M., and A. D. Krikorian, "*Eleutherococcus Senticosus* (Rupr. and Maxim.) Maxim. (Araliaceae) as an Adaptogen: A Closer Look," *Journal of Ethnopharmacology* 72, no. 3 (2000): 345–93.

12. Ernst, E., et al., eds., *The Desktop Guide to Complementary and Alternative Medicine: An Evidence-Based Approach* (Edinburgh: Mosby, 2001), 87.

13. Gaius Valerius Flaccus, "The Voyage of the Argo: The Argonautica of Gaius Valerius Flaccus," trans. D. R. Slavitt (Baltimore: Johns Hopkins University Press, 1999).

14. Germano, C., and Z. Ramazanov, *Arctic Root* (Rhodiola Rosea): *The Powerful New Ginseng Alternative* (New York: Kensington Books, 1999).

15. Gunther, R. T., trans., *The Greek Herbal of Dioscorides*, vol. 4, sec. 45, "*Rhodia Radis, Sedum Rhodiola*" (London: Hafner Publishing Company, 1968), 438.

16. Jellin, J., et al., *Pharmacist's Letter/Prescriber's Letter Natural Medicines Comprehensive Database*, 5th ed. (Stockton, CA: Therapeutic Research Faculty, 2003), 1167.

233

17. Kokoska, L., et al., "Screening of Some Siberian Medicinal Plants for Antimicrobial Activity," *Journal of Ethnopharmacology* 82, no. 1 (2002): 51–53.

18. Krendal, F. P., "Preparation Derived from Bio Mass of *Rhodiola Rosea* Tissue Culture," *Pharmacia* (Moscow), no. 5 (1989): 58–62.

19. Kurkin, V. A., and G. G. Zapesochnaya, "Chemical Composition and Pharmacological Properties of *Rhodiola Rosea Crassulaceae* (Review)," in Russian, *Chemico-Pharmaceutical Journal* 20, no. 10 (1986): 1232–44.

20. Lazarev, N. V., "Antiblastomogenic Medicinal Substances," in Russian, *Voprosy Onkologii*, in Russian, 11 (1955): 48–54.

21. Linnaeus, C. N., *Materia Medica. Liber I. De Plantis* (Stockholm, Laurentii Salvii, 1749), 168.

22. Linnaeus, C. N., *Örtabok* (Stockholm: Almquist and Wiksell, 1725), 127.

23. Magnusson, B., *Fägringar: Växter Som Berör Oss* [Beauty: Herbs that touch us] (Östersund, Sweden: Berntssons, 1992), 66–67.

24. National Pharmacopeia of the USSR, Rhodiola Rosea Rhizome and Roots, 11th ed. (Moscow: Medizina Press, 1998), 364–66.

25. Panossian, A., G. Wikman, and H. Wagner, "Plant Adaptogens: Earlier and More Recent Aspects and Concepts on Their Mode of Action," pt. 3, *Phytomedicine* 6, no. 4 (1999): 287–300.

26. Petkov, V., et al., "Pharmacological Investigations on *Rhaponticum Carthamoides*," *Planta Medica* 50, no. 3 (1984): 205–9.

27. *Pharmacopoea Svecica*, Homiae (Stockholm): Henrik Fougt, 1775.

28. Ramazanov, Z., and M. del Mar Bernal Suarez, *Effective Natural Stress and Weight Management Using* Rhodiola Rosea *and* Rhododendron Caucasicum (East Canaan, CT: ATN/Safe Foods Publishing, 1999).

29. Saratikov, A. S., and E. A. Krasnov, *Rhodiola Rosea Is a Valuable Medicinal Plant (Golden Root)* (Tomsk, Russia: Izdatelstvo Tomskogo Univ., 1987).

30. Saratikov, A. S., and E. A. Krasnov, "Stimulative Properties of *Rhodiola Rosea*," chap. 3 in *Rhodiola Rosea Is a Valuable Medicinal Plant (Golden Root)* (Tomsk, Russia: Izdatelstvo Tomskogo Univ., 1987).

31. Seifulla, R. D., *Sports Pharmacology Source Book* (Moscow: Mosovskaya Prauda, 1999).

32. Spasov, A. A., et al., "A Double-Blind, Placebo-Controlled Pilot Study of the Stimulating and Adaptogenic Effect of *Rhodiola Rosea* SHR-5 Extract on the Fatigue of Students Caused by Stress during an Examination Period with a Repeated Low-Dose Regimen," *Phytomedicine* 7, no. 2 (2000): 85–89.

33. Syrov, V. N., S. S. Nasyrova, and Z. A. Khushbaktova, "The Results of Experimental Study of Phytoecdysteroids as Erythropoiesis Stimulators in Laboratory Animals," in Russian, *Eksperimental'Naia i Klinicheskaia Farmakologiia* 60, no. 3 (1997): 41–44.

34. Udintsev, S. N., and V. P. Shakhov, "Decrease of Cyclophosphamide Haematotoxicity by *Rhodiola Rosea* Root Extract in Mice with Ehrlich and Lewis Transplantable Tumors," *European Journal of Cancer* 27, no. 9 (1991): 1182.

35. Wagner, H., H. Norr, and H. Winterhoff, "Plant Adaptogens," *Phytomedicine* 1 (1994): 63–76.

36. Weiner, M. A., and J. Weiner, "Ashwaganda (India Ginseng)," in *Herbs That Heal*, 70–72 (Mill Valley, CA: Quantum Books, 1994).

THE CHARM OF PROMETHEUS

37. Gunther, R. T., trans., *The Greek Herbal of Dioscorides*, vol. 4, sec. 45, "*Rhodia Radis, Sedum Rhodiola*" (London: Hafner Publishing Company, 1968).

Dioscorides of Anazarba in Cilicia was a surgeon to the Roman legions of Emperor Claudius when he wrote *De Materia Medica* in the 1st century A.D. This compendium of botanical medicines became the primary source of knowledge for herbalists for 1,500 years. It was first translated into English by John Gunther between 1652 and 1655 and included this note about *Rhodiola rosea*:

Rhodia radix [some call it Rodida] grows in Macedonia being like to Costus, but lighter, & uneven, making a scent in ye bruising, like that of Roses. It is of good use for ye aggrieved with headache, being bruised & layered on with a little Rosaceum, & applied moist to ye forehead, & ye temples.

38. Colchis civilization was formed from tribal confederations on the eastern shore of the Black Sea during the Bronze Age (1000–2000 B.C.). Archeologists have found extensive evidence of trade with Greece.

39. Gaius Valerius Flaccus, a Roman poet in the 1st century A.D., borrowed from Appolonius and wrote his own elaboration of *The Argonautica*.

40. Apollonius of Rhodes recorded the legend of Jason and the Golden Fleece in his 3rd-century B.C. epic poem *The Argonautica*.

41. The Golden Fleece has a basis in historical fact. In the legend, after crossing the Black Sea, the Argonauts traveled down the River Phasis (now the Rioni River). Mountain villagers in that area used sheepskins to trap gold dust in rivers flowing from the Caucasus Mountains. These gold-laden sheepskins were hung, dried, and beaten to shake loose the gold dust.

42. *Apollonius Rhodius: Argonautica*, book 2, lines 1245–50, ed. and trans. R. C. Seaton (Cambridge, MA: Harvard University Press, 1912), electronic edition, ed. Douglas B. Killings (1997), http://sunsite.berkeley.edu/OMACL/Argonautica (accessed January 20, 2004).

43. Medea was a priestess of the goddess Hecate. She became the instrument of revenge for the goddess Hera with the aid of Aphrodite. Athena and Hera decided to punish King Pelius after he killed a woman who had sought refuge at Hera's altar. The goddesses protected Jason on his voyage. Then Aphrodite sent Eros, the god of love, whose arrow drove Medea to fall in love with Jason so that she would protect him and return with him to Greece. The goddesses used Medea as their instrument of revenge to arrange the murder of Pelius. Medea persuaded the king's other daughters to kidnap him at night by promising to restore his youth with her magic. She then tricked them into killing, mincing, and boiling their own father.

44. Hecate, Queen of the Night, was supreme goddess in the heavens and the underworld. She favored her handmaiden, Medea, and taught her the use of herbs.

45. Folk remedies use *Rhodiola rosea* as a topical ointment or poultice as well as in liquid form for oral ingestion.

46. *Apollonius of Rhodes: Jason and the Golden Fleece*, trans. Richard Hunter, Oxford World's Classics (New York: Oxford University Press, 1993), 86.

47. Ibid., 95.

48. *Rhodiola rosea* grows in the high reaches of the Caucasus Mountains. It is a tough plant that survives high winds and freezing storms. When the pale root is cut, it has a dark sap and gives off the scent of roses. From each root may rise single, double, triple, or multiple stalks to a height of 12 to 24 inches (70 centimeters). It bears a flower the color of saffron.

CHAPTER 5

1. Baranov, V. B., "Experimental Trials of Herbal Adaptogen Effect on the Quality of Operation Activity, Mental and Professional Work Capacity," in Russian, Contract 93-11-615, Stage 2, Phase I, Moscow, Russian Federation Ministry of Health Institute of Medical and Biological Problems (IMBP), 1994.

2. Barker, A., R. Jones, and C. Jennison, "A Prevalence Study of Age-Associated Memory Impairment," *British Journal of Psychiatry* 167, no. 5 (1995): 642–48.

3. Bremner, J. D., et al., "Magnetic Resonance Imaging–Based Measurement of Hippocampal Volume in Posttraumatic Stress Disorder Related to Childhood Physical and Sexual Abuse—A Preliminary Report," *Biological Psychiatry* 41, no. 1 (1997): 23–32.

4. Bremner, J. D., et al., "MRI and PET Study of Deficits in Hippocampal Structure and Function in Women with Childhood Sexual Abuse and Posttraumatic Stress Disorder," *American Journal of Psychiatry* 160, no. 5 (2003): 924–32.

5. Bremner, J. D., et al., "MRI-Based Measurement of Hippocampal Volume in Patients with Combat-Related Posttraumatic Stress Disorder," *American Journal of Psychiatry* 152, no. 7 (1995): 973–81.

6. Brichenko, V. S., I. E. Kupriyanova, and T. F. Skorokhova, "The Use of Herbal Adaptogens with Tricyclic Antidepressants in Patients with Psychogenic Depression," in *Modern Problems of Pharmacology and Search for New Medicines*, ed. A. S. Saratikov (Tomsk, Russia: Izdatelstvo Tomskogo Univ., 1986), 58–60.

7. Crook, T. H., 3rd, and G. J. Larrabee, "Diagnosis, Assessment and Treatment of Age-Associated Memory Impairment," *Journal of Neural Transmission Supplementum,*33 (1991): 1–6.

8. Cummings, J. L., "Understanding Parkinson Disease," *JAMA: The Journal of the American Medical Association* 281, no. 4 (1999): 376–78.

9. Darbinyan, V., et al., "*Rhodiola Rosea* in Stress Induced Fatigue—a Double Blind Cross-Over Study of a Standardized Extract SHR-5 with a Repeated Low-Dose Regimen on the Mental Performance of Healthy Physicians during Night Duty," *Phytomedicine* 7, no. 5 (2000): 365–71.

10. De Deyn, P. P., et al., "Treatment of Acute Ischemic Stroke with Piracetam. Members of the Piracetam in Acute Stroke Study (PASS) Group," *Stroke; a Journal of Cerebral Circulation* 28, no. 12 (1997): 2347–52.

11. Engelhart, M. J., et al., "Dietary Intake of Antioxidants and Risk of Alzheimer Disease," *JAMA: The Journal of the American Medical Association* 287, no. 24 (2002): 3223–37.

12. Foley, D. J., and L. R. White, "Dietary Intake of Antioxidants and Risk of Alzheimer Disease," *JAMA: The Journal of the American Medical Association* 287, no. 24 (2002): 3261–63.

13. Gouliaev, A. H., and A. Senning, "Piracetam and Other Structurally Related Nootropics," *Brain Research. Brain Research Reviews*19, no. 2 (1994): 180–222.

14. Hoyer, S., "Oxidative Metabolism Deficiencies in Patients with Alzheimer's Disease," *Acta Neurologica Scandinavica. Supplementum* 165 (1996): 18–24.

15. Kessler, J., et al., "Piracetam Improves Activated Blood Flow and Facilitates Rehabilitation of Poststroke Aphasic Patients," *Stroke; a Journal of Cerebral Circulation* 31, no. 9 (2000): 2112–16.

16. Koivisto, K., et al., "Prevalence of Age-Associated Memory Impairment in a Randomly Selected Population from Eastern Finland," *Neurology* 45, no. 4 (1995): 741–47.

17. Krasik, E. D., K. P. Petrova, and G. A. Rogulina, "Adaptogenic and Stimulative Effect of Golden Root Extract," in *Proceedings of All Soviet Union Congress of Neuropathologists and Psychiatrists*, Sverdlovsk City, Russia, May 26–29, 1970, 215–17.

18. Mattson, M. P., and D. Liu, "Energetics and Oxidative Stress in Synaptic Plasticity and Neurodegenerative Disorders," *Neuromolecular Medicine* 2, no. 2 (2002): 215–31.

19. Petkov, V. D., et al., "Changes in Brain Biogenic Monoamines Induced by the Nootropic Drugs Adafenoxate and Meclofenoxate and by Citicholine (Experiments on Rats)," *General Pharmacology* 21, no. 1 (1990): 71–75.

20. Petkov, V. D., et al., "Effects of Alcohol Aqueous Extract from *Rhodiola Rosea L.* Roots on Learning and Memory," *Acta Physiologica et Pharmacologica Bulgarica* 12, no. 1 (1986): 3–16.

21. Saratikov, A. S., "Screening for Natural Central Nervous System Stimulants," in *Stimulants of the Central Nervous System*, vol. 1. (Tomsk, Russia: Izdatelstvo Tomskogo Univ., 1966) 3–23.

22. Saratikov, A. S., and E. A. Krasnov, "Clinical Studies of Rhodiola rosea," chap. 8 in *Rhodiola Rosea Is a Valuable Medicinal Plant (Golden Root)* (Tomsk, Russia: Izdatelstvo Tomskogo Univ., 1987).

23. Sastre, J., et al., "Mitochondrial Damage in Aging and Apoptosis," *Annals of the New York Academy of Sciences* 959 (2002): 448–51.

24. Shevtsov, V. A., et al., "A Randomized Trial of Two Different Doses of a SHR-5 *Rhodiola Rosea* Extract versus Placebo and Control of Capacity for Mental Work," *Phytomedicine* 10, no. 2–3 (2003): 95–105.

25. Spasov, A. A., et al., "A Double-Blind, Placebo-Controlled Pilot Study of the Stimulating and Adaptogenic Effect of *Rhodiola Rosea* SHR-5 Extract on the Fatigue of Students Caused by Stress during an Examination Period with a Repeated Low-Dose Regimen," *Phytomedicine* 7, no. 2 (2000): 85–89.

26. Spasov, A. A., V. B. Mandrikov, and I. A. Mironova, "The Effect of the Preparation Rodakson on the Psychophysiological and Physical Adaptation of Students to an Academic Load," in Russian, *Eksperimental'Naia i Klinicheskaia Farmakologiia* 63, no. 1 (2000): 76–78.

27. Stancheva, S. L., and A. Mosharrof, "Effect of the Extract of *Rhodiola Rosea L.* on the Content of the Brain Biogenic Monoamines," in French, *Medecine Physiologie Comptes Rendus de l'academie Bulgare des Sciences* 40, no. 6 (1987): 85–87.

28. Tritschler, H. J., L. Packer, and R. Medori, "Oxidative Stress and Mitochondrial Dysfunction in Neurodegeneration," *Biochemistry and Molecular Biology International* 34, no. 1 (1994): 169–81.

29. Vernon, M. W., and E. M. Sorkin, "Piracetam: An Overview of Its Pharmacological Properties and a Review of Its Therapeutic Use in Senile Cognitive Disorders," *Drugs and Aging* 1, no. 1 (1991): 17–35.

CHAPTER 6

1. Abidoff, M., et al., "Effect of *Rhodiola Rosea* and *Rhodiola Crenulata (Crassulaceae)* Root Extracts on ATP Content in Muscle Mitochondria," in Russian, *Biulleten' eksperimental'noi biologii i meditsiny* 136, no. 12 (forthcoming): 667–69.

2. Baranov, V. B., "The Response of Cardiovascular System to Dosed Physical Load under the Effect of Herbal Adaptogen," in Russian, Contract 93-11-615, Phase I and Phase II, Moscow,

Russian Federation Ministry of Health Institute of Medical and Biological Problems (IMBP), 1994.

3. Beauchaine, T., "Vagal Tone, Development, and Gray's Motivational Theory: Toward an Integrated Model of Autonomic Nervous System Functioning in Psychopathology," *Development and Psychopathology* 13, no. 2 (2001): 183–214.

4. Coyle, E. F., "Physiological Determinants of Endurance Exercise Performance," *Journal of Science and Medicine in Sport/Sports Medicine Australia* 2, no. 3 (1999): 181–89.

5. Porges, S. W., "The Polyvagal Theory: Phylogenetic Substrates of a Social Nervous System," *International Journal of Psychophysiology: Official Journal of the International Organization of Psychophysiology* 42, no. 2 (2001): 123–46.

6. Saratikov, A. S., *Golden Root (Rhodiola Rosea)* (Tomsk, Russia: Izdatelstvo Tomskogo Univ., 1974).

7. Saratikov, A. S., and E. A. Krasnov, *Rhodiola Rosea Is a Valuable Medicinal Plant (Golden Root)* (Tomsk, Russia: Izdatelstvo Tomskogo Univ., 1987).

8. Seifulla, R. D., *Sports Pharmacology Source Book* (Moscow: Mosovskaya Prauda, 1999).

9. Shevtsov, V. A., et al., "A Randomized Trial of Two Different Doses of a SHR-5 *Rhodiola Rosea* Extract versus Placebo and Control of Capacity for Mental Work," *Phytomedicine* 10, no. 2–3 (2003): 95–105.

10. Spasov, A. A., et al., "A Double-Blind, Placebo-Controlled Pilot Study of the Stimulating and Adaptogenic Effect of *Rhodiola Rosea* SHR-5 Extract on the Fatigue of Students Caused by Stress during an Examination Period with a Repeated Low-Dose Regimen," *Phytomedicine* 7, no. 2 (2000): 85–89.

11. Spasov, A. A., V. B. Mandrikov, and I. A. Mironova, "The Effect of the Preparation Rodakson on the Psychophysiological and Physical Adaptation of Students to an Academic Load," in Russian, *Eksperimental'Naia i Klinicheskaia Farmakologiia* 63, no. 1 (2000): 76–78.

CHAPTER 7

1. Baranov, V. B., "Experimental Trials of Herbal Adaptogen Effect on the Quality of Operation Activity, Mental and Professional Work Capacity," in Russian, Contract 93-11-615, Stage 2, Phase I, Moscow, Russian Federation Ministry of Health Institute of Medical and Biological Problems (IMBP), 1994.

2. Baranov, V. B., "The Response of Cardiovascular System to Dosed Physical Load under the Effect of Herbal Adaptogen," in Russian, Contract 93-11-615, Phase I and Phase II, Moscow, Russian Federation Ministry of Health Institute of Medical and Biological Problems (IMBP), 1994.

3. Bogatova, R. I., et al., "Avian Reproductive Function under a Combined Effect of Phytoadaptogens and Some Factors of a Space Flight," *Acta Veterinaria BRNO* 65, no. 1 (1996): 87–92.

4. Dudley-Rowley, M., "Deviance among Expeditioners: Defining the Off-Nominal Act through Space and Polar Field Analogs," *Human Performance in Extreme Environments* 2, no. 1 (1997): 119–27.

5. Foale, M., "NASA Oral Histories," R. Wright, C. Butler, and M. Davidson, interviewers, June 16, 1998, NASA, http://spaceflight.nasa.gov/history/shuttle-mir/people/oral-histories/foale.pdf (accessed August 15, 2003).

6. Kanas, N., "Psychosocial Factors Affecting Simulated and Actual Space Missions," *Aviation, Space, and Environmental Medicine* 56, no. 8 (1985): 806–811.

7. Kass, J., R. Kass, and I. Samaltedinov, "Psychological Considerations of Man in Space: Problems and Solutions," *Acta Astronautica* 36, no. 8–12 (1995): 657–60.

8. Khrunov, E. V., "Some Psychological and Engineering Aspects of the Extravehicular Activity of Astronauts," *Life Sciences and Space Research* 11 (1973): 91–103.

9. Kraft, N. O., T. J. Lyons, and H. Binder, "Group Dynamics and Catecholamines during Long-Duration Confinement in an Isolated Environment," *Aviation, Space, and Environmental Medicine* 74, no. 3 (2003): 266–72.

10. Long, M. E., "Surviving in Space," *National Geographic* 199, no. 1 (2001): 6–29.

11. Manzey, D., and B. Lorenz, "Human Performance during Spaceflight," *Human Performance in Extreme Environments* 4, no. 1 (1999): 8–13.

12. Polyakov, V. V., "The Use of a New Phytoadaptogen under Conditions of Space Flight," (abstract presented at symposium, Adaptogens: A New Group of Pharmacologically Active Substances Which Increase the Non-Specific Resistance of the Organism, Gothenburg, Sweden, November 4–5, 1966).

CHAPTER 8

1. Afanas'ev, S. A., et al., "Participation of Inducible Stress-Proteins in Realizing the Cardioprotective Effect of *Rhodiolae Rosea*," in Russian, *Biokhimiia* 61, no. 10 (1996): 1779–84.

2. Baranov, V. B., "The Response of Cardiovascular System to Dosed Physical Load under the Effect of Herbal Adaptogen," in Russian, Contract 93-11-615, Phase I and Phase II, Moscow, Russian Federation Ministry of Health Institute of Medical and Biological Problems (IMBP), 1994.

3. Brown, R. P., Gerbarg, P. G., and Ramazanov, Z., "*Rhodiola Rosea*: A Phytomedical Review," *HerbalGram*, no. 56 (2002): 41–52.

4. Kaplan, G. A., "Social Contacts and Ischaemic Heart Disease," *Annals of Clinical Research* 20, no. 1–2 (1988): 131–36.

5. La Rovere, M. T., et al., "Baroreflex Sensitivity and Heart-Rate Variability in Prediction of Total Cardiac Mortality after Myocardial Infarction. ATRAMI (Autonomic Tone and Reflexes after Myocardial Infarction) Investigators," *Lancet* 351, no. 9101 (1998): 478–84.

6. Maslova, L. V., and I. u. B. Lishmanov, "Accumulation of 99m-Technetium-Pyrophosphate and the Level of Cyclic Nucleotides in the Myocardium during Its Adaptation to Stress Damage," in Russian, *Patologicheskaia Fiziologiia i Eksperimental'Naia Terapiia*, no. 3 (1989): 53–55.

7. Maslova, L. V., I. u. B. Lishmanov, and G. N. Smagin, "Participation of Opioid Peptides in Regulating the Biosynthesis of Myocardial Protein during Stress and Adaptation," in Russian, *Voprosy Meditsinskoi Khimii* 37, no. 1 (1991): 63–65.

8. Mezzacappa, E. S., et al., "Vagal Rebound and Recovery from Psychological Stress," *Psychosomatic Medicine* 63, no. 4 (2001): 650–57.

9. Smirnov, A. V., et al., "Ecological and Physiological Problems of Adaptation," (proceedings, VII All-Russian Symposium, 1994), 254.

CHAPTER 9

1. Balog, P., et al., "Depressive Symptoms in Relation to Marital and Work Stress in Women with and without Coronary Heart Disease. The Stockholm Female Coronary Risk Study," *Journal of Psychosomatic Research* 54, no. 2 (2003): 113–19.

2. Bremner, J. D., et al., "Magnetic Resonance Imaging–Based Measurement of Hippocampal Volume in Posttraumatic Stress Disorder Related to Childhood Physical and Sexual Abuse—A Preliminary Report," *Biological Psychiatry* 41, no. 1 (1997): 23–32.

3. Bremner, J. D., et al., "MRI and PET Study of Deficits in Hippocampal Structure and Function in Women with Childhood Sexual Abuse and Posttraumatic Stress Disorder," *American Journal of Psychiatry* 160, no. 5 (2003): 924–32.

4. Bremner, J. D., et al., "MRI-Based Measurement of Hippocampal Volume in Patients with Combat-Related Posttraumatic Stress Disorder," *American Journal of Psychiatry* 152, no. 7 (1995): 973–81.

5. Brichenko, V. S., I. E. Kupriyanova, and T. F. Skorokhova, "The Use of Herbal Adaptogens with Tricyclic Antidepressants in Patients with Psychogenic Depression," in *Modern Problems of Pharmacology and Search for New Medicines*, ed. A. S. Saratikov (Tomsk: Izdatelstvo Tomskogo Univ., 1986), 58–60.

6. Centers for Disease Control and Prevention, "Web-Based Injury Statistics Query and Reporting System (WISQARS)," 2001, Centers for Disease Control and Prevention, http://www.cdc.gov/ncipc/wisqars (accessed August 12, 2003).

7. Goode, E., M. Petersen, and A. Pollack, "Antidepressants Lift Clouds, But Lose 'Miracle Drug' Label," *New York Times*, June 30, 2002, sec. A1.

8. Krasik, E. D., et al., *New Data on the Therapy of Asthenic Conditions: Clinical Prospects for the Use of Golden Root Extract (Rhodiola)* (Kemerov, Russia: Russian Academy of Medicinal Sciences, 1970), 298–300.

9. Solomon, Z., "The Impact of Posttraumatic Stress Disorder in Military Situations," *Journal of Clinical Psychiatry* 62, suppl. no. 17 (2001): 11–15.

10. Spasov, A. A., et al., "A Double-Blind, Placebo-Controlled Pilot Study of the Stimulating and Adaptogenic Effect of *Rhodiola Rosea* SHR-5 Extract on the Fatigue of Students Caused by Stress during an Examination Period with a Repeated Low-Dose Regimen," *Phytomedicine* 7, no. 2 (2000): 85–89.

11. Stimmel, G. L., "How to Counsel Patients about Depression and Its Treatment," *Pharmacotherapy* 15, no. 6, pt. 2 (1995): S100–S104.

12. World Health Organization, "The World Health Report 2001: Mental Disorders Affect One in Four People," World Health Organization, http://www.who.int/inf-pr-2001/en/pr2001-42.html (accessed August 8, 2003).

CHAPTER 10

1. Andrea, H., et al., "Association between Fatigue Attributions and Fatigue, Health, and Psychosocial Work Characteristics: A Study among Employees Visiting Physicians with Fatigue," *Occupational and Environmental Medicine* 60, supp. no. 1 (2003): i99–i104.

2. Blockmans, D., et al., "Combination Therapy with Hydrocortisone and Fludrocortisone Does Not Improve Symptoms in Chronic Fatigue Syndrome: A Randomized, Placebo-Controlled, Double-Blind, Crossover Study," *American Journal of Medicine* 114, no. 9 (2003): 736–41.

3. Cleare, A. J., "The Neuroendocrinology of Chronic Fatigue Syndrome," *Endocrine Reviews* 24, no. 2 (2003): 236–52.

4. De Vente, W., et al., "Physiological Differences between Burnout Patients and Healthy Controls: Blood Pressure, Heart Rate, and Cortisol Responses," *Occupational and Environmental Medicine* 60, suppl. no 1 (2003): i54–i61.

5. Gaab, J., et al., "Hypothalamic-Pituitary-Adrenal Axis Reactivity in Chronic Fatigue Syndrome and Health under Psychological, Physiological, and Pharmacological Stimulation," *Psychosomatic Medicine* 64, no. 6 (2002): 951–62.

6. Lin, T. Y., "Neurasthenia Revisited: Its Place in Modern Psychiatry," *Psychiatric Annals* 22, no. 4 (1992): 173–87.

7. Perski, A., et al., "Emotional Exhaustion Common among Women in the Public Sector," in Swedish, *Lakartidningen* 99, no. 18 (2002): 2047–52.

8. Reyes, M., et al., "Prevalence and Incidence of Chronic Fatigue Syndrome in Wichita, Kansas," *Archives of Internal Medicine* 163, no. 13 (2003): 1530–36.

9. Saratikov, A. S., and E. A. Krasnov, "Clinical Studies of Rhodiola," chap. 8 in *Rhodiola Rosea Is a Valuable Medicinal Plant (Golden Root)* (Tomsk, Russia: Izdatelstvo Tomskogo Univ., 1987), 216–27.

CHAPTER 11

1. Aires, V. V., et al., "In Vitro and in Vivo Comparison of Egg Yolk–Based and Soybean Lecithin–Based Extenders for Cryopreservation of Bovine Semen," *Theriogenology* 60, no. 2 (2003): 269–79.

2. Aitken, R. J., and D. Sawyer, "The Human Spermatozoon—Not Waving But Drowning," *Advances in Experimental Medicine and Biology* 518 (2003): 85–98.

3. Arlt, W., et al., "Dehydroepiandrosterone in Women with Adrenal Insufficiency," *New England Journal of Medicine* 34, no. 14 (1999): 1073–74.

4. Basson, R., et al., "Efficacy and Safety of Sildenafil Citrate in Women with Sexual Dysfunction Associated with Female Sexual Arousal Disorder," *Journal of Women's Health and Gender-Based Medicine* 11, no. 4 (2002): 367–77.

5. Berman, L., et al., "Seeking Help for Sexual Function Complaints: What Gynecologists Need to Know about the Female Patient's Experience," *Fertility and Sterility* 79, no. 3 (2003): 572–76.

6. Buvat, J., "Androgen Therapy with Dehydroepiandrosterone," *World Journal of Urology* 21, 5 (2003), 346–55.

7. Carson, C. C., "Erectile Dysfunction in the 21st Century: Whom We Can Treat, Whom We Cannot Treat and Patient Education," *International Journal of Impotence Research* 14, suppl. no. 1 (2002): S29–S34.

8. Castellini, C., et al., "Oxidative Status and Semen Characteristics of Rabbit Buck As Affected by Dietary Vitamin E, C and N-3 Fatty Acids," *Reproduction, Nutrition, Development* 43, no. 1 (2003): 91–103.

9. Chen, H., et al., "Male Genital Tract Antioxidant Enzymes: Their Source, Function in the Female, and Ability to Preserve Sperm DNA Integrity in the Golden Hamster," *Journal of Andrology* 24, no. 5 (2003): 704–711.

10. Clayton, A. H., "Female Sexual Dysfunction Related to Depression and Antidepressant Medications," *Current Women's Health Reports* 2, no. 3 (2002): 182–87.

11. Fink, H. A., et al., "Sildenafil for Male Erectile Dysfunction: A Systematic Review and Meta-Analysis," *Archives of Internal Medicine* 162, no. 12 (2002): 1349–60.

12. Graham, J. K., and R. H. Foote, "Effect of Several Lipids, Fatty Acyl Chain Length, and Degree of Unsaturation on the Motility of Bull Spermatozoa after Cold Shock and Freezing," *Cryobiology* 24, no. 1 (1987): 42–52.

13. Hampl, R., M. Hill, and S. L. Sterzl, "Immunomodulatory 7-Hydroxylated Metabolites of Dehydroepiandrosterone Are Present in Human Semen," *Journal of Steroid Biochemistry and Molecular Biology* 75, no. 4–5 (2000): 273–76.

14. Kubin, M., G. Wagner, and A. R. Fugl-Meyer, "Epidemiology of Erectile Dysfunction," *International Journal of Impotence Research* 15, no. 1 (2003): 63–71.

15. Nurnberg, H. G., et al., "Sildenafil for Women Patients with Antidepressant-Induced Sexual Dysfunction," *Psychiatric Services* 50, no. 8 (1999): 1076–78.

16. Nurnberg, H. G., et al., 2003, "Viagra (Sildenafil Citrate) Treatment of Serotonergic Reuptake Inhibitor–Associated Female Sexual Dysfunction" (poster presented at the International Consultation on Erectile and Sexual Dysfunctions, Paris, June 23–July 1, 2003).

17. Nusbaum, M. R., "Erectile Dysfunction: Prevalence, Etiology, and Major Risk Factors," *Journal of the American Osteopathic Association* 102, no. 12, suppl. no. 4 (2002): S1–S6.

18. Saratikov, A. S., and E. A. Krasnov, "The Influence of Rhodiola on Endocrine Glands and the Liver," chap. 6 in *Rhodiola Rosea Is a Valuable Medicinal Plant (Golden Root)* (Tomsk, Russia: Izdatelstvo Tomskogo Univ., 1987).

19. Shabsigh, R., et al., "Sexual Dysfunction and Depression: Etiology, Prevalence, and Treatment," *Current Urology Reports* 2, no. 6 (2001): 463–67.

20. Shaeer, K. Z., et al., "Prevalence of Erectile Dysfunction and Its Correlates among Men Attending Primary Care Clinics in Three Countries: Pakistan, Egypt, and Nigeria," *International Journal of Impotence Research* 15, suppl. 1 (2003): S8–S14.

21. Swan, S. H., et al., "Semen Quality in Relation to Biomarkers of Pesticide Exposure," *Environmental Health Perspectives* 111, no. 12 (2003): 1478–84.

22. Tan, R. S., and S. J. Pu, "The Interlinked Depression, Erectile Dysfunction, and Coronary Heart Disease Syndrome in Older Men: A Triad Often Underdiagnosed," *Journal of Gender-Specific Medicine: JGSM* 6, no. 1 (2003): 31–36.

23. Tran, D., and L. G. Howes, "Cardiovascular Safety of Sildenafil," *Drug Safety* 26, no. 7 (2003): 453–60.

24. Yousef, M. I., F. M. El-Demerdash, and K. S. Al-Salhen, "Protective Role of Isoflavones against the Toxic Effect of Cypermethrin on Semen Quality and Testosterone Levels of Rabbits," *Journal of Environmental Science and Health, Part. B—Pesticides, Food Contaminants, and Agricultural Wastes* 38, no. 4 (2003): 463–78.

CHAPTER 12

1. Beresford, S. A., et al., "Risk of Endometrial Cancer in Relation to Use of Oestrogen Combined with Cyclic Progestagen Therapy in Postmenopausal Women," *Lancet* 349, 9050 (1997): 458–61.

2. Eagon, P. K., personal communication, October 10, 2003.

3. Eagon, P. K., et al., "Evaluation of the Medicinal Botanical *Rhodiola Rosea* for Estrogenicity" (abstract, American Association Cancer Research, forthcoming).

4. Gerasimova, H. D., "Effect of *Rhodiola Rosea* Extract on Ovarian Functional Activity" (proceedings, Scientific Conference on Endocrinology and Gynecology, Sverdlovk, Russia, September 15–16, 1970), 46–48.

5. Giardina, E. G., "Heart Disease in Women," *International Journal of Fertility and Women's Medicine* 45, 6 (2000): 350–57.

6. Ingram, D., et al., "Case-Control Study of Phyto-Oestrogens and Breast Cancer," *Lancet* 350, 9083 (1997): 990–94.

7. Saratikov, A. S., and E. A. Krasnov, "The Influence of *Rhodiola* on Endocrine Glands and the Liver," chapter 6 in *Rhodiola rosea Is a Valuable Medicinal Plant (Golden Root) (Tomsk, Russia: Izdatelstvo Tomskogo Univ., 1987):* 180–93.

8. *Shumaker S. A., et al., "Estrogen plus Progestin and the Incidence of Dementia and Mild Cognitive Impairment in Postmenopausal Women: The Women's Health Initiative Memory Study: A Randomized Controlled Trial,"* JAMA: Journal of the American Medical Association 289, 20 (2003): 2651–62.

9. Vastag, B., "Hormone Replacement Therapy Falls out of Favor with Expert Committee," *JAMA: Journal of the American Medical Association* 287, 15 (2002): 1923–24.

CHAPTER 13

1. Bocharova, O. A., et al., "The Effect of a *Rhodiola Rosea* Extract on the Incidence of Recurrences of a Superficial Bladder Cancer (Experimental Clinical Research)," in Russian, *Urologiia i Nefrologiia*, no. 2 (1995): 46–47.

2. Bogdashin, I. V., S. N. Udintsev, and N. I. Suslov, "Effects of Rodiola Extract on the Cytotoxic Activity of Natural Killer Cells of the Liver, Spleen, Lungs and Small Intestine in Rats after Partial Hepatectomy," in Russian, *Biulleten' Eksperimental'Noi Biologii i Meditsiny* 110, no. 10 (1990): 409–11.

3. Boon-Niermeijer, E. K., et al., "Phyto-Adaptogens Protect against Environmental Stress–Induced Death of Embryos from the Freshwater Snail *Lymnaea Stagnalis*," *Phytomedicine* 7, no. 5 (2000): 389–99.

4. Dement'eva, L. A., and K. V. Iaremenko, "Effect of a Rhodiola Extract on the Tumor Process in an Experiment," in Russian, *Voprosy Onkologii* 33, no. 7 (1987): 57–60.

5. Duhan, O. M., et al., "The Antimutagenic Activity of Biomass Extracts from the Cultured Cells of Medicinal Plants in the Ames Test," in Ukrainian, *Tsitologiia i Genetika* 33, no. 6 (1999): 19–25.

6. Dvornyk, A. S., T. P. Pererva, and V. A. Kukakh, "Screening Substances Derived from Cultures of Medicinal Plants for Antimutagenic Activity in the *Escherichia Coli*–Bacteriophage Lambda System," in Ukrainian, *Tsitologiia i Genetika* 36, no. 2 (2002): 3–10.

7. Furmanowa, M., et al., "*Rhodiola Rosea* in Vitro Culture—Phytochemical Analysis and Antioxidant Action," *Acta Societis Botanicorum Poloniae* 76, no. 1 (1998): 69–73.

8. Glaser, R., et al., "Hormonal Modulation of Epstein-Barr Virus Replication," *Neurodendocrinology* 62, no. 4 (1995): 356–61.

9. Hoeg, O. A., *Vare Medicinske Planter* (Oslo: Det Best, 1984), 237.

10. Iakubovskii, M. M., et al., "The Activity of the Lipid Peroxidation Processes in the Mucosa of the Rat Small Intestine and Its Morphofunctional State under Acute Irradiation and the Administration of Combined Preparations Created on a Base of Highly Dispersed Silica," in Russian, *Radiatsionnaia Biologiia, Radioecologiia/Rossiiskaia Akademiia Nauk* 37, no. 3 (1997): 366–71.

11. Leonard, B., "Stress, Depression and the Activation of the Immune System," *World Journal of Biological Psychiatry* 1, no. 1 (2000): 17–25.

12. Salikhova, R. A., et al., "Effect of *Rhodiola Rosea* on the Yield of Mutation Alterations and DNA Repair in Bone Marrow Cells," in Russian, *Patologicheskaia Fiziologiia i Eksperimental'-Naia Terapiia*, no. 4 (1997): 22–24.

13. Spasov, A. A., V. B. Mandrikov, and I. A. Mironova, "The Effect of the Preparation Rodakson on the Psychophysiological and Physical Adaptation of Students to an Academic Load," in Russian, *Eksperimental'Naia i Klinicheskaia Farmakologiia* 63, no. 1 (2000): 76–78.

14. Udintsev, S. N., et al., "The Effect of Low Concentrations of Adaptogen Solutions on the Functional Activity of Murine Bone Marrow Cells in Vitro," in Russian, *Biofizika* 36, no. 1 (1991): 105–8.

15. Udintsev, S. N., S. G. Krylova, and T. I. Fomina, "The Enhancement of the Efficacy of Adriamycin by Using Hepatoprotectors of Plant Origin in Metastases of Ehrlich's Adenocarcinoma to the Liver in Mice," in Russian, *Voprosy Onkologii* 38, no. 10 (1992): 1217–22.

16. Udintsev, S. N., and V. P. Shakhov, "Decrease of Cyclophosphamide Haematotoxicity by *Rhodiola Rosea* Root Extract in Mice with Ehrlich and Lewis Transplantable Tumors," in Russian, *European Journal of Cancer* 27, no. 9 (1991): 1182.

17. Worcester, S., "Routinely Monitor Fatigue in Ca Patients," *Clinical Psychiatry News* (June 2003): 32.

18. Yaremenko, A., "Complex Treatment of Severe Infectious Diseases" (dissertation, I. P. Pavlov St. Petersburg State Medical University, 1998).

CHAPTER 14

1. Abidoff, M. T., "Synergistic Effect of *Rhodiola Rosea* and *Rhododendron Caucasicum* Herbal Supplement on Weight Loss in Healthy Female Volunteers: Placebo Controlled Clinical Study," (forthcoming), in Russian, Grant 77–1997. Moscow, 1997.

2. Abidoff, M. T., and M. Nelubov, "Russian Anti-Stress Herbal Supplement Promotes Weight Loss, Reduces Plasma Perilipins and Cortisol Levels in Obese Patients: Double-Blind Placebo Controlled Clinical Study," (proceeding, Stress and Weight Management at Russian Perestroika/Healthy Diet, June 1–3, 1997, Caucasian Republic of Dagestan, Russia).

244

3. Adamchuk, L. B., "Effects of Rhodiola on the Process of Energetic Recovery of Rat under Intense Muscular Workload" (dissertation, Izdatelstvo Tomskogo Univ., 1969).

4. Adamchuk, V., and B. U. Salnik, "Effect of *Rhodiola Rosea* Extract and Piridrol on Metabolism of Rats under High Muscular Load," (conference proceedings, Institute of Cytology of Russian Academy of Science, Moscow, 1971).

5. Isomaa, B., "A Major Health Hazard: The Metabolic Syndrome," *Life Sciences* 73, no. 19 (2003): 2395–2411.

6. Kohen-Avramoglu, R., A. Theriault, and K. Adeli, "Emergence of the Metabolic Syndrome in Childhood: An Epidemiological Overview and Mechanistic Link to Dyslipidemia," *Clinical Biochemistry* 36, no. 6 (2003): 413–20.

7. Ljung, T., et al., "Treatment of Abdominally Obese Men with a Serotonin Reuptake Inhibitor: A Pilot Study," *Journal of Internal Medicine* 250, no. 3 (2001): 219–24.

8. Saratikov, A. S., and E. A. Krasnov, "Effect of *Rhodiola Rosea* on the Central Nervous System," chap. 5 in *Rhodiola Rosea Is a Valuable Medicinal Plant (Golden Root)* (Tomsk, Russia: Izdatelstvo Tomskogo Univ., 1987).

9. Vicennati, V., and R. Pasquali, "Abnormalities of the Hypothalamic-Pituitary-Adrenal Axis in Nondepressed Women with Abdominal Obesity and Relations with Insulin Resistance: Evidence for a Central and a Peripheral Alteration," *Journal of Clinical Endocrinology and Metabolism* 85, no. 11 (2000): 4093–98.

CHAPTER 15

1. Andersen, R. E., et al., "Effects of Lifestyle Activity versus Structured Aerobic Exercise in Obese Women: A Randomized Trial," *JAMA: The Journal of the American Medical Association* 281, no. 4 (1999): 335–40.

2. Brown, R. P., P. L. Gerbarg, and P. R. Muskin, "Complementary and Alternative Therapies in Psychiatry," in *Psychiatry*, 2nd edition, eds. A. Tasman, J. Lieberman, and J. Kay (West Sussex, England: Wiley, 2003).

3. Pratt, M., "Benefits of Lifestyle Activity versus Structured Exercise," *JAMA: The Journal of the American Medical Association* 281, no. 4 (1999): 375–76.

4. Radak, Z., et al., "Exercise Preconditioning against Hydrogen Peroxide–Induced Oxidative Damage in Proteins of Rat Myocardium," *Archives of Biochemistry and Biophysics* 376, no. 2 (2000): 248–51.

5. Strong, C., "Brain Mapping Pinpoints Adverse Effects of Minor Sleep Loss in Children," *Neuropsychiatry Reviews*, September 2003, 20–21.

6. Winnicott, D. W., "The Theory of the Parent-Infant Relationship," *International Journal of Psycho-Analysis* 43 (1962): 238–39.

INDEX

Underscored references indicate boxed text.

other names for, 73
overview, 73–74
side effects, 74
as true adaptogen, 57
Emotional energy drains, <u>44</u>
Emotional energy enhancers, <u>46</u>
Emotional reactions, changing, 32–33
Empathy
low RSA and, 29
sensitive stress response systems and,
30
Endocrine/metabolic system, 18
Energy. *See also* Building blocks of
energy; Fatigue
adaptogens for boosting, 59
aging and, 177–78
assessing regularly, importance of, 45
cellular production of, 9–10
constant need for, 4, 6
crisis, 11, 15–16
depletion, oxygen free radical
damage and, 14–15
drains, <u>44</u>, 47
enhancers, <u>46</u>, 47
imbalance, examples of *Rhodiola
rosea*'s effect on, 7–9
laws of balancing, 42–46
maintaining
methods for, 40–41
quiz for self-assessment, 39–41
oxygen free radicals and decline in, 10
pervasiveness of, in the human body,
6
Rhodiola rosea as enhancer, 47
as sign of good health, 20
spending more than you have, 3, 6, 9
stress/energy imbalance, diseases and,
17–18
supplements purchased to increase, 5
understanding needed for balanced
life, 21

Enhancers, energy, <u>46</u>, 47
Environmental stressors, 22
Epinephrine
adaptogens for guarding against
excessive, 59
damage from chronic exposure to,
16–17
as neurohormone, 12–13
released by adrenal medulla, 24
stress response system and, 12–13,
24
Erectile dysfunction (ED), 163–65
Estrogenic effect and cancer, 181
Exam periods for students, <u>195</u>
Exercise
for building energy, 215–17
erectile dysfunction and lack of, 163
as key to weight loss, 200
minimum needed, 216–17
perimenopause and, 178
stress response and, 216
Exhaustion phase of stress response,
25–26, 59
Extracts of *Rhodiola rosea*, buying,
67–68

F

Fatigue, 149–61
adrenal burnout, 159–61
burnout, 3, 16, 149
case studies, 150–51, 152–53, 155,
156, 157–59
cortisol levels and, 160
defined, 152
depression and, 155–56
examples of *Rhodiola rosea*'s effect
on, 7–9
exhaustion phase of stress response,
25–26, 59
gender and, 149

MPPA (mono- and polyphenolic acids) formula. *See* ADAPT formula
Multivitamins, 214
Muscle-building, *Rhodiola rosea* for, 104–5
Muscle mass loss, 16–17, 112
Muscular dystrophy, 108, 109
Musculoskeletal system diseases, 18

N

Naps, 43
Nausea, from *Rhodiola rosea*, 70
Nerve cells
    damaged by chronic stress, 25
    protected by *Rhodiola rosea*, 11
Network theory of aging, 64
Neurasthenia, 131–32, 153–54. *See also* Fatigue
Neuroendocrine systems, 5
Neurohormones. *See* Stress hormones
Neurological system diseases, 17–18
Neurotransmitters, hippocampus damage from, 25, 85
Neurotrophic factors, 35
Nitrates (angina medications), 164
Norepinephrine
    adaptogens for guarding against excessive, 59
    damage from chronic exposure to, 16–17
    as neurohormone, 12–13
    production stimulated by *Rhodiola rosea*, 87
    released by locus coeruleus, 23, 24
    stress response system and, 12–13, 23–24
Normalizing action (adaptogen criterion), 57
Nuts in high-energy diet, 212

O

Obsessive-compulsive disorder, 142–43, 147–48
Omega-3 essential fatty acids, 214
Optygen sports formula, 112
Oriental ginseng. *See Eleutherococcus senticosus*
Oxidative damage, 10, 11
Oxidative stress, 10
Oxygen free radicals
    antioxidants as defense, 186
    beneficial actions of, 10
    calorie restriction and, 35–36
    damage done by, 10, 85
    energy depletion and damage by, 14–15
    mitochondria damaged by, 15

P

Panax ginseng
    for head trauma, 96
    long-term effects of, 73
    other adaptogens compared to, 76–81
    other names for, 72
    overview, 72–73
    side effects, 72–73
    as true adaptogen, 57
Parasympathetic nervous system (PNS)
    activated by ADAPT formula, 106
    function of, 13, 15–16, 26–27
    heart rate and, 29
    impaired by stress response system, 13
    rest needed for, 16
    underactivation, illness due to, 17
    vagus nerve and, 27–28

Research
double-blind, placebo-controlled
studies, 90
growing body of, for *Rhodiola rosea*,
4–5
pharmaceutical companies and,
179–80
on *Rhodiola rosea* and
antistress and stimulant effects,
92–93
cancer protection and treatment,
187–88, 192–93
depression, 131–32
DNA repair, 187–88
heart function, 124–26
infection protection and healing,
194–95
mental performance, 88–91
muscle-building, 105
physical performance, 107–8
safety, 180–83, 182
weight loss, 202–4
studies of
ADAPT formula, 88, 106,
117–18, 120, 121
adaptogens by Soviets, 53, 56–58,
105–6
Eleutherococcus senticosus, 73
mental performance, 87–91
Panax ginseng, 72
Rhaponticum carthamoides, 74
Schizandra chinesis, 74
Withania somnifera, 75
Resistance, nonspecific (adaptogen
criterion), 57
Resistance phase of stress response, 25,
59
Resistance to stress, building, 34–36
Respiratory sinus arrhythmia (RSA),
28–29, 29
Reticular activating system, 87

Rhaponticum carthamoides, 57, 74,
76–81
Rhodiola species other than *rosea*, 68
Rhododendron caucasicum, 202–4
Rituals and routines, 221
RNA, *Rhodiola rosea* and, 105
Rosavins, 67
RSA (respiratory sinus arrhythmia),
28–29, 29
Russian ginseng. *See Eleutherococcus
senticosus*

S

Safety of *Rhodiola rosea*, 63, 180–83
SAM-e, 97, 214
Saunas, 34–35
Schizandra chinesis
in ADAPT formula, 88, 106
other adaptogens compared to,
76–81
overview, 74–75
side effects, 75
as true adaptogen, 58
Secondary amenorrhea, 176
Second Wind sports formula, 112
Seeds in high-energy diet, 212
Selective serotonin reuptake inhibitors.
See Antidepressants
Self-assessment. *See* Quizzes
Self-blame, understanding and, 21–22
Serotonin, 87
Sertraline (Zoloft). *See* Antidepressants
Sexual dysfunction, 162–73. *See also
specific forms*
antidepressants and, 166
case studies, 165–67, 169
depression and, 166–67
difficulties discovering source of,
162–63
erectile dysfunction (ED), 163–65

space missions and, 113–22

stress/energy imbalance, diseases and, 17–18

understanding needed for balanced life, 21

Stress/energy balance

imbalance and diseases, 17–18

laws of energy balancing, 42–46

quizzes for self-assessment, 37–42

Stress hormones. *See also* Cortisol; Epinephrine; Norepinephrine

adaptogens for guarding against excessive, 59

damage from chronic exposure to, 16–17

heart rate and, 123–24

neurohormones defined, 12–13

Stressors

bodily defense mechanisms for, 23

chronic, damage from, 26

defined, 22

duration of, effects of stress and, 24

extreme, damage from, 25–26

fatigue caused by, 154–55

forms of, 22–23

inability to control, 45–46

positive events as, 23

psychological reactions to, 26

quiz for zeroing in on, 38–39

Stress response system

activation by brain, 23–24

adaptogen criteria and, 58

aging and, 19

autonomic nervous system and, 12

changing reactions, 31–33

elasticity of, 35

energy depletion in, 11

energy regulation by, 13–14

exercise and, 216

fight-or-flight response, 12–14, 30–31

heart affected by, 123–24

long-term triggering of, 13

mild stress as beneficial for, 34

overactive

balancing, 42

quiz for assessing, 41–42

sensitivity and, 30–31

overview, 23–24

parasympathetic nervous system impaired by, 13

phases of stress response, 25, 59

as primitive adaptation, 101–2

quizzes for self-assessment, 37–42

sensitivity, quiz for self-assessment, 41–42

stabilizing, 33

sympathetic nervous system triggering of, 12–13

underactive, in criminals, 31

Stroke, calorie restriction and, 36

Students, vulnerability to infection, 195

Studies. *See* Research

Sudarshan Kriya Yoga (SKY), 222–24

Suicide in youth, depression and, 133–34

Supplements

for building energy, 214–15

side effects of energy-enhancing, 5

Sympathetic nervous system (SNS)

heart rate and, 29

HPA axis coordination with, 12

overactivation, illness due to, 17

stress response system and, 12–13, 23–24

Synergy sports formula, 111, 112

T

Tablets of *Rhodiola rosea*, buying, 68–69

Tadalafil (Cialis), 164

Printed in the United States
by Baker & Taylor Publisher Services